For My Donor

20 Years and Counting

By Mark Watson

To all those who support organ donation

Acknowledgements

The process of writing this book was always going to be a painful one, but little did I realise just how much impact it would have on my life. Throughout the whole journey I have been faithfully supported by the one person closest to me despite the enormous ramifications it had on that relationship. My then partner and now close friend Jennifer has encouraged me, calmed me in moments of panic and has been at my side through every twist and turn the story took. Without her none of the following pages would have been written, so I owe a huge debt of gratitude for all that she has put up with. Thank you.

Many more people have helped me along the way. Bec and Willow helped ease my passage back into the transplant community and provided guidance and encouragement that kept me going when it felt like the end would never be reached.

In writing the book my main concern was the impact on the donor families. Thanks goes to Sally for reviewing some of my words and reassuring me that the book would have a positive impact on those involved in the painful side of organ donation.

My close friends Sean and Sarah helped me by attending events with me that helped shape a number of chapters. It is always fun spending time with your friends and I'm lucky to enjoy such great company. I also have Yomi to thank just for being there to hear my moaning when things were not going to plan.

Final editing of the book was assisted by my good friend Heather. This was completed as a favour to me and I'm grateful for her input and also her kind words.

Thanks also go to all my other friends who offered their support throughout the last 15 months. This has come both from personal conversations and through many conversations with fellow transplant patients on Twitter. Every single comment has encouraged me to keep going.

Finally thanks go to my mother. Sometimes being a mother is a thankful task, especially when both your sons have suffered from ill health. I wouldn't be here without her and I will always be grateful for that.

Contents

The Story of Claire Sylvia   6

Cellular Memory   20

Test 1 - Heightened Fears   35

The 1994 World Cup   50

Reflections   63

Test 2 - The Slope   77

The Ten Year Letter   93

The Birthday   105

Test 3 - Fiddle This   115

Heroes, Villains and the Gift of Life   127

Welcoming the Intruder   140

Test 4 - Boyz II Men   157

Depression   169

A Question of Sex   181

Test 5 - The Gay Test   195

Meeting Your Donor Family   208

The Case for the Opposition   222

Test 6 - A New Love   236

Who Is My Donor?   253

The Longest Night   269

Appointment with Destiny   282

Meeting the Family   295

The Story of Claire Sylvia

"It is infinitely better to transplant a heart than to bury it to be devoured by worms."

Christian Barnard (Cardiac Surgeon who performed the world's first successful human-to-human heart transplant)

Today is a Wednesday. As with most Wednesdays, I find myself working through several insurance projects, none of which stimulate any enthusiasm, nor engage my attention. I am bored. Taking a break, I open the inbox to my personal emails and reveal a new message that instantly lifts my spirits. There is an email from a lady named Amara Cohen. I have never spoken with Amara but a few days previously I had made tentative contact via the internet, after reading a book written by her mother. Amara's mother is Claire Sylvia.

During 1996, Claire Sylvia was a medical celebrity. She had received one of the very first combined heart and lung transplants at the Yale New Haven Hospital in Connecticut USA, eight years earlier. She had written and launched an autobiographical account of her health experience, covering her remarkable journey from miserable ill health, to consenting to and undergoing pioneering, lifesaving surgery.

At this time in modern history, organ transplantation was becoming a more frequent occurrence. Bookshelves were filling with the amazing recounts of patients detailing their own roads to recovery. Every single one inspirational in its own way but none so unique or different that it would create a media frenzy, or bring the event from the health sections towards to the front pages of the news agenda.

Ms Sylvia, however, had an original perspective. Just five days after her operation, journalists and reporters had been invited into Yale New Haven Hospital, proud of their recent endeavour, to speak to the first heart and lung recipient. During the press conference which was necessarily held in the intensive care unit, one eager reporter asked of Sylvia, "Now that you've had this operation, what do you want, right now, more than anything?"

I can imagine the reporter at the time, asking the question to elicit a decent front page headline quote. Sylvia's response was a surprise to herself and everyone else present.

"To tell you the truth, right now, I'd die for a beer."

In this moment, Sylvia felt that she could identify a change in herself that was more than just replaced organs, to pump blood and breathe air into her body. She had just recognised an experience she would view as 'cellular memory', a scientifically unproven idea that each individual cell in our bodies contains unique markers that reflect our personality and character.

Like I'm sure the majority of people reading the article, I quickly dismissed the story as that of someone with new age and spiritual beliefs and not something to be taken seriously. After all, I'd lost my brother to illness as he waited urgently for a heart transplant, and then later going on to receive a donor heart myself after discovering we both had a genetic heart condition.

I was still in grief and trying to understand everything I had gone through physically and mentally through those first painful years, and I certainly wasn't ready to explore a possibility of something unusual going on with my transplanted organ.

But something has nagged at me down the years and, like most transplant recipients, I'm both eternally grateful and curious to know more about this special person that enabled me to go on living. Maybe I'd undergone some changes too? Perhaps there was some part of me celebrating this amazing gift by enjoying some of the small things my donor did?

As a transplant patient, I've generally kept myself separate from other transplantees. I've not been one for the forums, help groups, or even just building a few like-minded friendships. I've not been someone who has always been writing to, or trying to meet my donor family. In part it's because I find the more I talk about the subject, the more anxious I get about my own health, and also because I haven't wanted to be defined by my transplant. I'm happy to be defined by my love of Norwich City, my guitar playing, my slightly bumpy relationship history or my volunteering, just not my new heart.

But 19 years have passed and that's already 14 more than I expected to get after the operation (survival rates are just one issue you quickly become aware of post-transplant). I'm now more settled about myself, my brother and thinking of my donor, so maybe now is a good time to see if there is something in 'cellular memory'. Certainly Amara's response not only gives me encouragement, but she also offers hope of putting my mind finally at ease with what these last two decades have thrown at me.

"If you can, try and find out about your donor, if nothing else it will bring closure to you and possibly the donor family. I still receive holiday cards from the mother of my mother's donor."

Without precedent and lacking a guide book on finding donors and how to deal with the mind-boggling array of thoughts and emotions that immediately fill my mind, the only question I have is "where to start?"

The notion that I may have inadvertently inherited characteristics from my donor is overwhelming. Not something my friends can easily understand. Most of them look at me in disbelief, as though I had said aliens had landed from another planet.

My partner, Jennifer, is more enthusiastic and helps me to begin thinking through all the implications of starting this unusual journey.

My mind moves immediately; what of the donor families? What would their responses be, presented with the information that their deceased loved-ones' organs might have essentially altered the character of their recipients. The last thing I *ever* want to do is show insensitivity towards this wonderful group of people. Making a decision to donate a loved-ones' organs must be one of the most difficult and traumatic in the world. At the time of huge stress and emotional trauma, a family is asked to consider the lives of others too, before letting their beloved relative pass. Nobody could ever truly measure what these people mean to us transplantees.

It does seem truly odd that an organ such as a heart could hold memories from the life before: tastes, people, and places. I guess my real concern is for the feelings of the donor families, if this were true. I imagine cellular memory to be more like a photograph. The grainy picture I look at of my brother shows him at around ten years of age, sitting with a small fishing rod, knees bent leaning towards the river, looking out more in quiet thought than in hope of a catch. It is very real and comforting for me, seeing him there. A real memory of a happy, innocent time when we couldn't have known or even imagined the trauma that lay ahead. This is how I imagine my heart to have captured those memories. In my chest, the heart beating is still very much a part of me, it is *not* my donor. Yet maybe it has a sense of where it was before.

Claire Sylvia's book made a dramatic impact, creating confusion for what this meant to transplanted patients and the moral dilemmas it posed. Useful for book sales, less so for people's peace of mind and for the general public who always worry about what it would mean to be a donor. There were genuine concerns about what this new aspect would do to the already limited supply of donor organs.

Dr. Marc Lorber, Head of the transplant unit at Yale New Haven Hospital, spoke of these worries in an article published in the London Sunday Times prior to Sylvia's book launch.

"If transplant surgery becomes linked in some way, either emotionally, subliminally or otherwise, to the supernatural, it could be highly problematic for the future of transplant surgery. It has the potential to generate negative feelings about organ donation. Despite tremendous success of transplant surgery, we still only have a consent rate of about 50%, so we have a long way to go before the notion of organ donation is generally accepted. I have obviously heard the stories being circulated by Claire Sylvia, but it should be made clear that the concept of cellular memory has no medical foundation. To the best of anyone's knowledge it does not exist

So could everything that Claire Sylvia reported just be the good-natured intentions of a transplant recipient wanting to get closer to the person that had unintentionally saved her life?

Sylvia is not like me. She was a self-confirmed believer in a spiritual world, (though this means different things to different people, of course) and had always felt that the world was not the stark black and white contrast that medical science and her doctors had spelled out to her. She already felt there was more meaning to be interpreted than most. Once she was officially added to the transplant waiting list, she was the type of person that did research and being open minded, was ready for something as mysterious as 'cellular memory'.

Sylvia had spent much her life dealing with ill health despite being a professional dancer, and finally, in 1983, she was diagnosed with primary pulmonary hypertension, a disease which causes blood vessels in the lungs to collapse. As her health worsened she became house and wheelchair bound, requiring oxygen just to complete the simplest of tasks. Being finally placed on the transplant list in those early days must have been both a sign of hope, but equally a huge step into the unknown.

Eventually, when her call came, Sylvia showed great bravery and calmness, as she was rushed to hospital with her daughter at her side, arriving and meeting the surgeons who were to perform the first heart and lung transplant at the hospital.

Almost immediately after the surgery, Sylvia began to experience changes and thoughts that alerted her to think something significant was happening on a psychological level; more than her doctors could understand. After all, they had never had a transplant themselves, so her experience and opinion put her in a unique position and also, very new territory.

A small amount of information was given to Sylvia, three days after the operation. The organs had come from an 18 year old boy who had been killed in a motorcycle accident. As someone who had always paid attention to and analysed her dreams, it was quickly noted that a mysterious stranger began to feature regularly when she returned home. The first time this happened was exhilarating for her and in her book, she describes her dream;

"I'm in an open, outdoor place with grass all around, it's summer. With me is a young man who is tall, thin, and wiry with sandy coloured hair. His name is Tim – I think it's Tim Leighton, but I'm not sure. I think of him as Tim L. We're in a playful relationship, and we're good friends.

"It's time for me to leave, to join a performing group of acrobats. I start to walk away from him, but I suddenly feel that something remains unfinished between us. I turn around and go back to say goodbye. Tim is standing there watching me, and he seems happy when I return.

"Then we kiss. And as we kiss, I inhale him into me. It feels like the deepest breath I've ever taken, and I know that Tim will be with me forever."

Anyone reading this account might find the experience a little too intense for comfort. Having been through a transplant operation, I read her words and don't acknowledge it as an experience I have shared but I do recognise the deep emotional bond and gratitude that Sylvia must have been feeling towards this unknown person who had saved her life.

As the weeks and months go by, Sylvia experiences other strange changes. She develops a craving for chicken nuggets and green peppers; she starts to walk with a more masculine gait. She is drawn to different women than she was before and feels an abundance of youthful energy.

After being told by the hospital staff that they could not provide her with any information about her donor, Sylvia eventually took the decision to try and track down this person who she has been calling Tim. With a friend she begins scrolling through old newspapers on the local libraries microfiche, ultimately being shocked to find the report of an eighteen year old boy being killed on a motorbike the day of her own transplant. The name of the boy was: Tim.

Liking beer after an operation is one thing, I think we all are all in an odd place those first few weeks, but for Sylvia to have dreamt the correct name of her donor seems astounding to me. Probably a huge coincidence, but nonetheless astounding.

Sylvia went on to meet her donor's family and during that emotional first acquaintance, she was able to establish a few other details about Tim. He drank beer, he had a taste for chicken nuggets (they were found on him at the time of his accident) and he was well known for being restless, with energy to spare. These were all in line with changes Sylvia had experienced. It all seemed to prove that her hypothesis was correct; a transplanted organ consisted of *more* than just tissue. The heart isn't just a basic pump.

The organs also carried around memories, in each and every single cell. These memories could be interpreted by a patient in tune with their body.

Not everyone was ready to accept this idea, just as I wasn't as I struggled with my own recovery. Indeed her doctor, on first hearing what Sylvia was suggesting, had told her to "act normal", and "stop all this touchy-feely stuff and get on with your life." If that sounds harsh, then the audience that greeted Sylvia and her new donor family on the Phil Donohue show was much more scathing, the story of her dream inhaling Tim, was met with laughter.

But time has passed and many more transplantees have reported the kind of changes that Sylvia was brave enough to speak about. Regardless of your belief in cellular memory, you can't hide from the fact that undergoing a transplant is a psychologically difficult process. Sylvia was certainly 100% genuine about what she believed, and her gratitude and love for her donor family is not in question, and to me that's the most important thing.

"I definitely believe the heart transplant gave my mother new emotions and likes and dislikes, but they did fade over time once the heart settled into who she was. When she had a kidney transplant 10 years later, from a boyfriend, it didn't have the same effect as the heart did. Maybe because she knew the donor so well or because it was a kidney and not a heart."

So maybe even Sylvia began to doubt the changes she had felt so strongly, or, as she reported in her book she just settled into this new person she had become.

One thing is sure though, Claire Sylvia left a legacy. She opened the door to other patients to express their beliefs that they had undergone strange changes after receiving new organs. She also showed those people on the waiting list that a transplant was not something to be scared of, that these donated organs could "breathe new life" into someone that was near to death. Far from having a life full of complications, you could go on to enjoy a life that was richer and more enjoyable than before. She was an inspiration to many.

No matter how inspired or encouraged I am, I can't help but contemplate the sensibility of doing the same. Should I put myself through the emotional trauma of trying to understand if I too, have been though personality changes due to my own donor? I reflect on Amara's comments about closure for her mother and I read back a passage from Sylvia's book that moved me to tears.

Sylvia has just been invited into the house of her donor family; it was an exhausting and highly emotional first meeting. She hadn't known what to expect, with both of her donors parents showing little emotion when she had first called them on the phone. At first Sylvia declines the invitation, already emotionally drained and with a long journey home ahead of her.

"Well okay," June, her donor's mother replies, "I've just made a little cake to go with some coffee."

With this kind, final offer, Sylvia accepts and steps back inside the house. June disappears and finally returns with a huge cake that has been decorated with a single word.

"WELCOME"

We all want to belong, and we all want to know where we have come from. A little part of me has been through its own journey, and has a history with a whole different family.

I really don't know if 'cellular memory' exists, but maybe I need to be 'welcomed', and to say my thanks to my wonderful donor.

Cellular Memory

"Science knows it doesn't know everything; otherwise, it'd stop. But just because science doesn't know everything doesn't mean you can fill in the gaps with whatever fairy tale most appeals to you."

Dara Ó Briain (stand up comedian and host of "Dara Ó Briain's Science Club")

I've been firing off emails most of the day in an attempt to find out more about cellular memory and its impact on transplant recipients. I actually start to feel a bit claustrophobic as though my chest is tightening and the walls are closing in on me. I start to wonder if this impact is psychosomatic or if my donor is trying to tell me that I'm getting closer to this mysterious secret.

A lot of the research seems to be anecdotal, with many stories similar to that of Claire Sylvia, and then a few studies on things such as neurones, that as yet I don't profess to understand.

Today I watched an interesting documentary by the Mindshock team on Channel 4 called "Transplanting Memories", in which the makers spoke to both Claire Sylvia and a few other transplant patients who shared their stories. Most of the medical information came from Dr Paul Pearsall and Dr Rollin McCraty who spoke about the heart having a miniature brain that could hold memories, allowing it to know when to pump and pass information back to the brain. Interestingly though, the documentary also spoke to renowned transplant surgeon Professor Sir Magdi Yacoub of Imperial College, London. Whilst not accepting the notion of cellular memory, he stated "whenever you come with a wild idea, if you like, it needs to be refuted, and if we can't refute it maybe there is something there."

So who are Dr Paul Pearsall and Dr Rollin McCraty, and what studies have they conducted? Is there something I can learn for my own experiment?

Sadly Dr. Pearsall passed away in 2007 following a spell in hospital, but from his own website there is a long list of fairly impressive achievements. He was a licensed clinical neuropsychologist, clinical professor at the University of Hawaii, and on the Board of Directors of the Hawaii State Consortium for Integrative Health Care. The list of achievements includes an award by the Oxford Biographical Society as one of the 1000 most influential scientists of the 20th Century. He is credited with producing ground-breaking research on heart transplant recipients receiving the memories of their donor. He has appeared on Oprah several times.

Through a web search I come across Pearsall's original research paper;

CHANGES IN HEART TRANSPLANT RECIPIENTS THAT PARALLEL THE PERSONALITIES OF THEIR DONORS

Dr Pearsall is evidently a man who has already made up his mind about the existence of cellular memory and the paper highlights ten cases to prove the point. Whilst some can easily be passed off as coincidence, others are quite staggering in the amount of detail the recipient seems to know about their donor.

I don't know how I felt after reading these stories. I feel fairly upset and also a little bit guilty. It's clear that for the majority of the recipients the connection is an important and emotional one. On a personal level, I've always felt a bond to my donor without being able to put a name or face to that feeling. The sense of loss I have for my brother Adrian is replicated in the thoughts I feel for my donor. I feel loss there too. Maybe that's just me transposing my emotions on to the heart that beats harder when I think about it, or maybe there is truly something there.

The guilt comes from the overriding realisation of how important all this is to the donor families. It's their one last piece of connection and obviously they want to believe something is there. I feel as though I've maybe let my donor family down, maybe I haven't allowed them that connection.

There is no real conclusion in the paper but it finishes by trying to prompt debate, "The present findings are reported with the hope that they will stimulate future research to examine the hypothesis seriously". I wonder if my efforts would be considered "serious". Maybe not. At least their study was of 74 transplant patients. Mine is only of one, myself, but at least I'm looking at it as a doubter. I want some real proof.

The stories listed do at least seem to have some consistency in the types of changes the transplant patients have gone through. I try grouping them so I can start to assess where I may have been affected.

Having a feeling towards a certain name

Changes in favourite foods

Sexual preference and increased libido

Shows traits typical of the opposite gender

Musical taste

Recognising music not previously heard

Recognition of donor and family

A feeling of disappointment that I have failed to achieve these markers starts to fill my head. After all these years, it is really hard to remember any changes in my behaviour. Any draw towards any names may have long since passed; I don't think my food or sexual preferences have passed. I know I don't like nuts but what about my taste buds?

I also feel as though the research didn't really investigate what else could have caused some of these changes in the patients, after all the whole process is a very emotional and stressful one. In the first few days the vast quantities of drugs produce a shock to the system and can leave you hallucinating and disorientated. In the long term the amount of tablets a patient takes can leave you with so many side effects it's hard to get back to who you were pre-transplant.

I do some quick sums. I've been a transplanted for 19 years now and I've probably averaged around 18 tablets a day in that time. Sometimes a lot more, sometimes a little less, so that's around 125,000 tablets. Some people find it hard taking an antibiotic, so imagine the changes from taking that little lot. I imagine the drugs in a pile. I imagine the cost. I remind myself the joys of living within a national health system. Thank you NHS.

Every transplant patient's medication will be different, and I'm not sure how typical mine is, but there will always be drugs to prevent rejection which work by suppressing the immune system. Other drugs will be there to help the transplanted organ work as well as it can within its new host body.

This is my current list of medication, and what I think it does for me. Apologies to any doctors who might be reading, in particular my own. It feels a bit of a test, but rest assured even if I get the reason wrong at least I'm taking them.

Sirolimus - this is my main rejection medicine, the little tablet that keeps me alive.

Prednisolone - a steroid that also helps rejection. Doesn't make me a world class athlete.

Clopidogrel - kind of like aspirin and thins my blood a little.

Allupurinol - because for some reason other things give me gout. Ouch. This prevents it.

Atorvastatin - to reduce the cholesterol that is raised by my rejection medicine.

Amiloride - helps keep my blood pressure under control, or at least I think it does.

Candesartan - also for blood pressure. Maybe I have too many of these?

Hydrocortisone - another steroid but this might make me a world class athlete.

Bumetanide - a diuretic that helps me get rid of fluid the only way the body knows how.

Ranitidine - prevents stomach ulcers that may develop from too many tablets!

I feel quite queasy having just written the list, so the effects of taking them will be huge. I take a look through all the leaflets that are included in the small boxes of tablets, to see if I can find the clues about changes in personality.

Confusion and hallucinations, changes in the way things taste, feelings of high mania or moods, seeing or hearing things that do not exist, changing how you act, increased appetite, worsening of schizophrenia, changes in behaviour, increase in hair growth, loss of appetite, decreased desire for sex, inability to maintain an erection, anorexia, sexual difficulties, breast enlargement, changes in personality.

Of course this is a small selection of the side effects listed. One mentioned is "heart failure", but reassuringly the leaflet advises "if any of the side effects get serious, please tell your doctor or pharmacist". I make a mental note to pick up the number of my local pharmacist and check for any signs of heart failure that could be serious.

I always wonder why side effects have to be negative in nature, always leaving the patient to weigh up the pros and cons of taking the medication provided to them. You never seem to find that the tablets may 'increase your tolerance to jazz', provide an 'ability to speak French' or make your penis a 'more desirable size for sexual pleasure'.

The drugs that we take and their side effects clearly could be one answer to the question of why transplant patients are reporting personality changes. Other aspects, such as the knowledge of names or the physical recognition of donor families cannot be explained by side effects. There is something more intrinsic; but how on earth would muscle tissue be able to remember a name? I really struggle to remember people's names, as it is, (I always attribute this to a side effect of medication), so how on earth would my heart be able to do a better job than my brain? Are there other factors at play?

One idea put forward to counter the claims of cellular memory is that of "hospital grapevine theory". This suggests that, even whilst unconscious, transplant patients pick up on discussions that may have taken place, within their locality, about their donor.

All transplant hospitals take donor confidentiality extremely seriously, and it would be a matter of real concern if they were to discover a doctor or nurse breaking this ethical code. As a patient I am allowed to contact my donor family should I wish, but the transplant clinic will hold the donor family details and will only pass on the letter on my behalf. Unless there is a specific request from the family, and my doctors know it is something I would be receptive to, I will never find out anything more than a rough age and sex.

So far, the cases I have found are limited when you consider the number of transplants worldwide. There were around 3000 transplants, for all organs, in the UK alone during 2011 (with over 7600 on the waiting list) so if there are only a handful of reported cases it is possible there could have been some minor breaches of confidentially that lead to some recipient knowledge.

My confidence in the professionalism of my transplant clinic is such that I have no doubt that any donor details wouldn't have been discussed in my presence. I did, however, have an experience of "grapevine theory" that would show how this theory might hold.

During my inpatient stays in both intensive care and high dependency units, I listened and responded to instructions. Considering I neither listen nor respond to commands now, it just shows how drugged up I must have been. Or maybe you need to be a nurse. I felt a great sense of care and warmth to those looking after me. It was only for a relatively short period but I was in the hands of others, in a life threatening situation. I quickly learned to trust and relax into dependency towards the professionals around me.

Much later, after a good few weeks spent recovering in the normal wards, my mother spotted a nurse walking along the corridor towards us. "Look who it is", my mother said, and I looked at this heavily pregnant lady, struggling to think if I had ever met this person at all. As soon as there was a "hello", everything changed and her voice took me straight back to feeling of being cared for and comforted. My brain could instantly recall the sounds and words that were spoken to me during those difficult first few days, even if I had no recollection of what this kind nurse looked like. I knew her name.

Of course it would be lovely to be able to thank that nurse now, but her name has now since left me (again, it's surely the medication to blame) and I'm sure after many transplant operations, she has also since forgotten me. All the same, thank you.

It starts to feel more and more like there are logical answers to some of the reported findings, yet whilst being a sceptic, I don't want it to just end here, closing the book on this idea of holding donor memories. Part of me wants to think there is some emotional as well as physical connection, after all, my life and that of my donor are tied together in a way very few people are, and I still have no knowledge of that person.

Some of the changes, such as musical taste, knowing songs and the recognition of a member of the donor family can't be answered by either side effects of drugs or hospital grapevine theory, so I still think I need to test the theory myself.

All the examples I've discovered so far could be explained, and that possibly the recipients knew something about their donor already. I'm clear that the only knowledge I have is that my donor was 33 and male. I know nothing more than that.

Through the experiment I hope to build up a mental picture of my donor both physically and in their tastes or desires. Once I have established my own thoughts about my donor, I aim to try and find out more about them and see if anything matches, hinting that the possibility of 'cellular memory' truly exists. It will also help me get closer to my donor, something I'd love to do at this point in my life.

I start trying to think through how my experiment might work:

I shouldn't attempt to find out anything about my donor until the experiment is complete.

The tests should include the majority of my senses, specifically my tastes, sexual preference and musical choices.

Tests should be based on things I know I didn't like pre-transplant, to gauge if I feel differently about them now.

I should try and build up a profile of the character traits I think defines my donor.

It's been 19 years since my transplant and it's hard to remember the "me" that came before the operation. Much of who I am has been shaped by experiences gained as an adult. We all go through phases. I used to wear a shell suit, like lots (well it felt like lots) of people in the 80's. I'd certainly hate that now, so how am I to know what's been potentially changed by my donor, and what's been changed by my life experiences.

I try and think what I was like as a child and a teenager. It's not an easy process when you have already lost the sibling that would tell you every negative trait you have in an instant. So instead I turn to a pile of my old photographs.

There's the first picture of the baby me, being cradled quite expertly by my Nan out in the garden of their home. I'm frowning, dressed in a white knitted top suitable for a girl and looking down to where Adrian remains firmly and safely on the ground.

Another shows a fairly handsome, yet nervous child sitting on a blue, three wheeled trike, my red shiny shoes reaching for the ground and waiting for the photo to be taken so I can go back to my favourite method of transport. Walking.

Running through dozens of these early pictures it becomes obvious I was a very timid child, scared of just about everything - although it could be I loved all the things I did as a child, maybe I just didn't like a camera pointing at me. There's me scowling with an ice cream, with my cousin Sarah; looking like I'm going to cry because of the size of conker I'm presenting to the taker of the photo; rubbing my eyes in disgust because I've been made to sit in a deck chair that has clashed with the stripy trousers I'm wearing.

Later photos show me smiling nervously as I'm photographed appearing out of a stone, slate tiled public toilet. I'm dressed in a 90's Adidas shell suit and everything about this picture seems to be hugely embarrassing.

Finally I come across something that makes me lose the smile that's been spreading across my face as I reminisce about childhood times. This photo shows me in the same nineties shell suit, proudly smiling into the afternoon sunshine, my arm around my mother, the shadows long across the spring grass. My mother is holding a cheque to a rather formal looking man, dressed in a grey, double-breasted suit. In his hand is a small electronic device aimed at helping those awaiting transplant. This is Papworth Hospital, just after Adrian's death, and as yet I'm unaware that I too have something wrong with my heart, that I will be one of those patients in need of the device we have come to fund.

I put the pictures down.

Test 1 - Heightened Fears

"You're so happy and grateful, but you know there is another family out there who is sad on that day, because when I take the steps, those are his lungs."

Dottie O'Connor (cystic fibrosis patient and lung transplantee who climbs a different mountain each year in memory of her 37-year-old mountain climbing donor).

In my early years I'd visited Paris many times. It had been, until my operation, my only trips abroad. I'd recently gone through all the photographs of my youth and amongst them were the faded blue skies of Paris framed by lush, green foliage. The Eiffel Tower's iron structure dominates the image, barely able to squeeze in its 6x4 inch borders. Yet, despite the trips, there isn't one picture looking down at the panoramic views the Tower offers tourists.

Fear has played a large part in my life and a fear of heights has always been a fairly debilitating and limiting experience. Part of the reason for not going abroad was a fear of flying. My anxiety of what goes up must come down, generally more quickly the latter rather than the former.

I wanted to see if fear had been a big factor in my donor's life? Were they as frightened or anxious about heights as I had been? Would I now be able to enjoy that view from the top of the Eiffel Tower?

Other transplant patients had made positive strides from the changes they had experienced and it was my hope I could feel just some part of that. Dottie O'Connor, of Massachusetts, had suffered from cystic fibrosis until she had a lung transplant. Heights had always been something more daunting than joyful, but after her operation she began making a pilgrimage up a different mountain each year in memory of her donor. Dottie was to learn that her donor was a 37 year-old mountain climber.

"I almost feel like he's climbing with me, because when I take the steps, those are his lungs."

Dottie has taken her experience and gone on to win Gold and Silver medals in track and field at the US Transplant Games. It's a great tribute to her donor, so surely I should be able to scale the small heights of the Eiffel Tower.

It's June and the trip was now just a few days away. I'd booked to go to Paris in January, mainly because I like to enjoy more foreign trips now (maybe that's something my donor liked more than me) and in part because it allowed me to travel on Eurostar, avoiding the plane journeys I endured rather than enjoy.

My partner Jennifer always likes to plan these things out, to know what she will be doing and when, and whilst I'm more of a free spirit, I do like to find an event or two to ensure we have some fun whilst we are there. I'd already managed to book us some time at the Paris Open, watching some of the minor matches on the outside courts, and a trip using the Batobus on the Seine. Part of me felt no need to book anything for the Eiffel Tower, it was going to be a big part of the journey, but it's always there and from memory there never seems to be a huge amount of people around, unlike London's main tourist attractions.

In a moment of boredom I clicked on the link to the Eiffel's main booking page, and selected a day when I thought we would have time to go up, "no tickets are available for your chosen day" came back the reply. Frantically I scanned the small calendar on the screen that seemed to suggest the only times available would be when we were already on the Eurostar train returning home. Was this fate trying to tell me something, or just bad timing that would mean I'd have to shelve my plans to try and understand my donor more?

I emailed Jennifer and gave her the bad news. I don't often use emoticons, but this felt like an appropriate moment for a sad, un-smiley face. To be truthful, I felt a little bit relieved. It's hard work testing something you're scared of, and scarier trying to assess if there really is something to this whole cellular memory thing.

I was just starting to accept that it wasn't meant to be when an email from Jennifer popped up in my inbox, "I can get one for 1:30". This seemed odd. The website seemed very sure of itself when I looked earlier. It had never suggested I "go away and think about it" or "ask someone else to make the booking and I'll see what I can do". I immediately jump back into the booking site, select my date again and sure enough there it is, availability at

1:30. I hardly skip a beat as I select two tickets, punch in my card details and download my printable tickets. It's on. I'm going up the Tower in just five days time.

Since my transplant I have travelled more extensively and so I have become used to flying. I've also found myself in some pretty high places, including the top of the Empire State Building. I was scared in the lift when going up again last August, but I can't remember a sense of panic coming over me as I stood at the top and stared down at the little yellow ant like cabs hurtling about the streets below.

The day after, though, two men had been shot dead right outside the building at the exact time we had been standing there the day before. I immediately felt that this was some sort of sign, and I should stay away from the things I fear. Heights are scary and it's probably only me that rightly acknowledges that. It reaffirmed my fears.

It's a Tuesday morning in Paris, and considering how the summer has been so far, it's an amazingly bright, blue-sky day with the temperature in the mid-twenties. The morning so far has been spent discussing the merits of single or block metro tickets, and having a polite argument with the charming French lady at the Batobus station. After many attempts at speaking French it became obvious that she didn't think my pre-planning was pre-planned enough. Finally, she relented and we got to enjoy the view from the calm waters of the Seine.

Up until now we have only seem glimpses of the top of the Eiffel Tower as it pierces through the top of Paris's many fine buildings and bridges. Although visibly large, it still seems like a postcard, or picture staring out from a newspaper report. It's only as we come around the corner on the Batobus that I see the Eiffel Tower again, in full view, for the first time in over twenty years. It's huge, and backdropped against the pure blue sky it reminds me of just how my photo looked back in my old album.

I look nervously at this old structure, the sunlight blazing not only over the edge of its peak, but through the beams and bouncing off the glass of the old lift as it makes its way slowly down the Tower's shaft. The Empire State Building kept its workings hidden, it felt solid and of stone, a straight forward shape that cocooned you from the views until you stepped outside to wonder just how high you'd gone. This was different, everything was outside. You were going to feel the journey up, and it felt old.

It's now 12:00 and so far we haven't discussed my thoughts or feelings about my donor, we are just happily taking photographs like the rest of the tourists that seem to number a few hundred. We're all looking for that same snap, and what with the Facebook and twitter generation, many are trying to make it look like they are holding the Eiffel Tower up with their bare hands. Fools I think, as I take yet another picture of blue sky and iron Eiffel. We find the spot where my picture was taken as a 20 year old. It's hard to believe what has happened in all that time, yet this spot has stood here relatively unchanged.

After a healthy dollop of hot dog in baguette (I know, how French), we wander over to the area designated for pre-booked tickets to assess if we are in the right place. I pass over my paperwork whilst remembering the long debate I had with the Batobus lady. Everything is in order, but as it is 1:05 we are told to come back in 20 minutes when we will be let into the area for the Eiffel Tower's lifts. We walk over to the edge of the square and take a seat on the curb to people watch and soak up the sun.

As I breathe out what appears to be a fairly relaxed breath, out of the corner of my eye I begin to notice three army-type figures a few metres away. All of them are in military fatigues and carrying automatic rifles, which is something I'm not used to seeing. I don't mention them, thinking to myself that the more I normalise the situation and don't react to it, the less chance I'll have of setting off some irrational thoughts.

"Look at them" says Jennifer, "I wonder what's going on?"

I hadn't wanted to think that anything was "going on". I had wanted Jennifer to say something like "oh, them again, they're always here for photos." As it is she has punctured my bubble, now thoughts of the Empire State Building killings are going through my head. How should I keep away from my fears? I mention to Jennifer the Norwegian mass killer, Anders Breivik, and suggest that dressing as the military would be a good way to conduct an attack. She agrees. I look back at the soldiers, and they turn away and head over to the crepe stall. Soon they disappear from sight and the discussion turns to my feelings.

"Are you excited?"

"I think so", which, on reflection suggests the complete opposite.

"How do I know which bit of me wants to do it and which bit doesn't?"

"Well are you being ruled by your head or by your heart?"

It seems a simple question, but it's one I find hard to work out. Part of me doesn't feel the need to do this. I know what's up there will look exactly like what's down here, only further away. Maybe that's my head saying "no". I do want to go up though, but partly because I need to find out how I feel when I'm there. I'd feel I had let my donor down if I didn't at least try.

The time has come to head back to the pre-booked area. We are the only ones there and despite it being a little early we are immediately waived through. We walk straight down past the line of walk up visitors, "Suckers!" I say to myself. What follows are the now common airport style security checks as we pass through x-ray machines for our back packs and metal detectors for ourselves. Before we know it we are standing in front of the first lift, which opens within what feels like seconds. A man on a stool beckons us in, and I find myself up the corner with a window in front and to the side of me. I feel relaxed, knowing we are only going up to the second floor.

Suddenly we are moving and as I look out, everything is disappearing much quicker than I imagined. The angle of the lift disorientates me and I feel a wave of panic starting to hit me in the chest and swim up my face. I lock tight onto the bars of the lift as Jennifer just smiles happily, enjoying the ride. As the lift stops the only things preventing me from pushing through all the tourists in front of me is the fact I'm still clutching the lift. A space appears, I move through it and onto the deck of the second floor. I can't go near the edge. There is no possibility of me falling, but everything feels unsteady beneath my feet. If I leave the comfort of the Eiffel's main frame I feel I will panic. No forget that. I am panicking.

If my donor is loving this, I clearly am not. I'm not even close to the top of the tower and already I feel worse than I ever did on the Empire State Building. Maybe it was the fact I could see out, as we travelled up in the lift, but right now I know I'm not going to be able to go any further.

"Stand by the telescope" Jennifer encourages me.

It should be easy, but each step feels like one step closer to the abyss. I reach out and clutch the golden object in front of me. Jennifer takes a picture of a man closing his eyes to look through a magnifying lens.

After a few minutes things begin to settle and I start to wander round the four sides of the tower, being careful to only push past people on the inside of the walkway. The views from here are incredible, and I know I'm fortunate to have such a clear blue day where you can see for miles all around. I look back down the gardens to where I was standing to replicate that picture of twenty years ago. I imagine the young me looking back to see the older version standing on the second floor and wonder what he might think. I try and see if anything feels familiar. Has my donor stood on this spot and looked out beyond? It's hard to imagine, but it reminds me why I'm doing this.

"Are you ready to go to the top?" Jen enquires.

"I don't know"

"Well if you don't I'm going anyway"

I run through my head if it will be harder to go up with company, or stay down here alone amongst the happy, secure, head-for-heights people.

"OK let's go"

The queue for the second lift is long and windy. Like all queuing systems it is roped and designed to make you move four-foot forward by walking twenty-foot horizontally to where you want to go. When we were at base level we were special, we were pre-booked, winners in the lift lottery. Now at the second level we are all part of the same class, no special treatment and the waiting time will only add to my frazzled nerves. Once more we try to work out what is driving me to do this. Is it my donor cheering me on in the knowledge that this is a heart that loves heights? Is it fear of letting my donor down and failing in some small way? Does it just not want to let Jennifer down?

I try to add some humour, as is normally the case when I am at my most frightened.

"They don't know we've got a cheap deal" I say nervously.

"What do you mean?" Jennifer's response has a hint of confusion, rather than intrigue.

"We've only paid for two tickets and there are three of us going up."

Jennifer smiles. I can tell my gallows humour has not quite hit the mark.

Within 15 minutes we are handing over our tickets again and from this spot I feel more secure, tucked within what feels like the belly of the tower. It's harder to see the views, and all I can spot is a few people standing, waiting for the next lift to come down. A door opens, and before I am ready a crowd of people are pushing me into the tight, cramped space of the lift. I'm not happy, but as the doors close I shut my eyes and hope that when I open them again I'll be safe.

"Nearly there," Jennifer whispers.

"Liar," I think.

It seems to take ages, but in the safety of my own darkness I feel much happier than when we were in the first lift. Then it was a shock, this time I'm beating the system. Fear is locked outside unable to find its way in through my eyelids. We stop. It takes a few seconds, but there is a jolt, a clunk, and we're there. I open my eyes to see people staring into the lift like cats staring into a goldfish bowl. The door opens the other side and we step out into the inner sanctum of the top of the tower.

From here all you can see is grubby windows framed by black, graffiti etched walls. It's hardly the nicest looking entrance, but it feels secure and as though you are not really part of the outside world. I look up and see a sign saying "Sommet" that points up a short flight of stairs. I'm pulled by my own desire to reach the top, so I rush up and out into the open air, leaving Jennifer trailing behind me.

I still feel wobbly, but I'm there and the views are unreal. Actually the views feel not dissimilar to the ones on the second floor, but the sense of achievement makes me look at them with a new wonder. Jennifer asks me if it feels like I should be here, and it does. It's a surreal feeling but I know this is something I can do, that a bit of me isn't as scared as the old me. In the past I could only look up and wonder how people could be so relaxed at being so high and now I was part of that club, but it felt like I have been part of that club for a while now. Those fears not quite as intense or debilitating as before.

I can feel my donor's heart pounding. Is it adrenaline fuelled by fear or excitement? My sense is that it's excitement and the only fear is what's being driven by my head. In the past my head would have ruled my heart, but clearly my donor is more dominant than me, pushing me on to new, ahem, heights.

We make our way round the top and I look for the champagne bar that was mentioned on the website. In truth it reminds me more of a kiosk at a football ground than some salubrious bar, but the one thing less in common is that it's pricing is even more extortionate at 12 euros a glass.

"Should I celebrate, it is for my donor after all?" I ask Jennifer.

"It's up to you. You could have a slushy at the bottom"

I love icy slush. My head wins this time, and so does my pocket.

I take some final pictures to commemorate the event, forming my hands into a heart shape to show that I'm up here with my donor heart. It's a proud moment, and that feeling calm all fear and makes the thought of the lift back down a much easier one. After a short wait we are beginning the journey down the shaft of the Tower and I look up through the glass panel to see the top slowly shrinking in size. We step from one lift immediately into another and I'm breathing easily and laughing as we begin our final descent to the bottom of the Tower again. I walk from the lift with the easy stroll of a Tower regular.

Looking back at the Eiffel Tower whilst enjoying the rewards of an orange slushy (apparently the lemon one I wanted was iced up), it has lost all of the threat it seemed to pose before and just has a majestic, almost retro beauty to me. I take a few pictures of the people looking at us from the safety of the second floor, and some more of the lift going up and down and marvel at how I could allow myself to be inside it.

Before Paris is done for the day, we head over to Notre Dame Cathedral. I'm not someone who is at all religious, but I understand the importance of religion to those who are, and I also believe in celebrating the memory of loved ones. Normally in a church or cathedral I'll light a candle to my brother, but today it's for my donor. I look at the small candle flickering away in the beauty of hundreds of other such memories, and thank myself that there are such wonderful donor families out there. It's been a good day.

The 1994 World Cup

"As the doctors say, I shouldn't have survived, I'm working towards my comeback. If I can, I will, and if not, no problem, I'll carry on with my family life."

Eric Abidal (professional footballer with France and Monaco and liver transplant recipient)

It's a cloudy day in California. Roberto Baggio, the Italian playmaker walks slowly up to the penalty spot, his hair tied back in his trademark ponytail, the blue shirt of his country loosely hanging outside of his shorts. As he places the ball on the spot, 94,000 fans inside the Rose Bowl hold their breath; another couple of billion people remain glued to their television screens. Baggio can't seem to decide between placement or power and ends up smashing the ball high into the Pasadena sky and providing the moment their opponents have been waiting for. Brazil are the 1994 World Cup champions.

One day later and the party can still be heard in Rio de Janeiro, whilst closer to home a family is about to make a decision that will change their lives and ultimately change the life of a complete stranger.

The day had started fairly routinely for a Monday morning, I was working full time in my job at an insurance company and in general I was feeling relatively healthy. In fact it was pretty hard to believe my life was slowly slipping away as only months earlier I was happily playing football and hockey on a regular basis, so how come I needed this operation. Although it had been a while since my assessment at Papworth Hospital, where a decision is made to accept you for organ transplant, I had only officially been on the list for ten days. I can hear the screams of protestation from the transplant community; it almost felt like I hadn't earned my badge. Like the fifth Brazilian penalty taker, I'd been put on the list but never had to take my spot kick, or to feel the pressure. I'd won the World Cup but had I deserved it?

Most people can wait months or years for a transplant, and in fact nearly half of those waiting will end up dying before an organ becomes available, so whilst I was still getting used to the idea of being on the list, I didn't really expect anything to happen very quickly. I had been called a couple of times during the month long World Cup from my transplant co-ordinator checking on my health and ensuring I didn't have any coughs and colds. I had always been very clear, "Don't call me yet, I'm enjoying the World Cup, just wait until it's finished". Well now it had finished, and as I set about sorting out the morning's post I was happily reflecting on the previous night's final.

I carried a mobile phone with me at all times. As someone on the list you need to be contactable and ready to leave at a moment's notice, and in those days mobile phones were the status symbols of the upwardly mobile businessman. I certainly wasn't "upwardly mobile", more horizontal and exhausted. My business acumen had thus far been restricted to selling painted rocks back to the very same children that had painted them in the first place, when I was eight years old. Like most of the elderly generation today, I still wasn't used to having a mobile phone, and on that Monday morning I was walking around without actually having it switched on.

As I busied about my work (to be fair, I probably ignored my work and just chatted to whatever colleague was closest by), I was still in a fairly relaxed mood. Then it began. A colleague called me over, saying she had a call for me. It was my transplant co-ordinator. They had been trying to contact me on my mobile but without success. They had some important news, they had got a donor.

I wasn't quite sure what to say. What is the etiquette in these situations? Should you say 'thank you', shout as though you have Tourette's or hug the first person within range? I just stood there, put the phone down and casually told my colleagues I would be on my way.

First of all though, I wanted a coffee and to call my partner Becky to let her know it was time to go. Within a few moments the phone went again. The transplant co-ordinator was back, "Just a quick reminder" she said, "don't have anything to eat or drink". I put the coffee down first, and then the phone.

My bag was already packed, and my car was parked in the car park of our office building. There was the option of travelling by ambulance, but part of me was excited by the idea that this was my one opportunity in life to speed as fast as I could in my car. It's a rare event that someone could be stopped by the police and then when asked what the rush is, can respond "I'm just on my way for a heart transplant officer".

Soon enough Becky and I were speeding along the Norfolk countryside, Becky making calls to my mother and other family members to let them know what was happening. It was surreal, and I've never felt more focused on driving my car. There was no point thinking about what lay ahead, this was just a time to get on with it.

On arrival we were greeted by the transplant co-ordinator and shown to a private room where a few tests could be carried out to check on my current condition, and so I could begin getting myself prepared for the operation. Up on the wall of the room I noticed a picture in a frame. It was of a small girl kneeling and praying by the side of her bed. It was the same picture my mother also had, and for some reason it made me feel as though everything was going to be alright. Next a razor was handed to me. I know these surgeons have standards but I didn't think I needed to make myself presentable for an operation. I had to shave off some of my body hair. My legs, is that enough? My chest? Arms too? That as well? This is really too much. I've only had to shave hair from that region once before, and it was the growing back that caused more distress than the original removal.

The time was steadily moving into the evening, and if you've ever been in hospital for an operation you'll know that not much happens after normal working hours. On that night though, there almost appeared to be a crackle of anticipation around the place. It's as though everyone knows a transplant is going to happen, and I'm the minor celebrity in this weird scenario. Surgeons have been called in, anaesthetists readied and a team on standby just waiting to receive this strangers heart that's going to save my life.

After what seems a long wait, the transplant co-ordinator makes an appearance back in the room, everything with the heart is healthy, it looks good and is suitable for transplantation. It's on. At that moment I felt my old heart begin to shiver and race, suddenly it all felt a little real. Maybe I'd been fooling myself, but somehow it was still so far off before, now it was really going to happen.

Before I know it I'm being wheeled through a chain of corridors. It's always an odd sensation looking up at the ceiling as lights flash by and doors open and swing shut behind you. There are no other scenarios where I am wheeled flat on my back anywhere. In some ways we should do more of it. I'd particularly like to not have to leave my bed in order to get to work, but right now I feel caught between the feeling of being terrified and that of being a rock star on his way to the stage.

Finally I'm in the small room where the anaesthetist will do his work. With any normal operation I would already have left any family behind on the ward, but here in the room with me is my mother and Becky. To start with there is silence, and through the doors we can all see the theatre lights looking down, spotlighting the operation table that is obscured by the doors between us.

The anaesthetist speaks. I can't remember his words but I know they are comforting and he strokes my hand with more affection than the rest of us dare show. He asks if we want to say anything before he puts me under, and it's at that point I finally break down and lose control of my emotions. Suddenly I'm caught up in the finality of what we are saying, that this might actually turn out to be the end.

My final words are "I'll see you later". To this day I never say "goodbye" to anyone. It's too final. I prefer "see you later", although that can confuse the supermarket checkout staff that are only putting through your groceries.

There isn't really time to get composed, but after calming a little and kissing both Becky and my mum I start counting down from 10 as the anaesthetic starts to kick in. I don't remember how far I got, but now everything was out of my hands.

The next room I saw was one I'd seen a few times before. I'd been asked if I wanted to take a look inside the intensive care unit the week I'd had my assessment for going on the list. I hadn't. I'd made it to the door and the emotion of it all was too much for me to bear. There was nothing overly frightening through the doors, just two beds, maybe a bit more equipment than your average hospital bed, but nothing too out of the ordinary. The only thing holding me back was memories. The memory of this room, with my brother Adrian in the bed, slowly losing his battle with life. Would you want to go back? I didn't, but now the situation was forced. I was in my own battle. In that same room.

My memory of the first day is pretty hazy. I am told I flitted in and out of consciousness, and that I was always very distressed when I came round. My body and mind was fighting to escape that room, but physically I wasn't ready for it and I was kept sedated to keep me a little calmer. I've always hated operations. It seems something that even my unconscious mind knows I'm a bit of a coward when it comes down to it.

Most transplantees I speak to talk of how amazing it felt to be able to breathe and feel the beating of this new heart inside of them. I just felt like crap. Every part of my body felt like it had been spun round inside a washing machine at high speed and then dumped back inside of me. Maybe it's because I had been fairly fit? All the tests showed I was dying, but I had been physically active and with energy. I hadn't experienced heart attacks or being unable to breathe. I'd felt fairly ok, now was much worse.

But was I experiencing any changes? One of the most defining moments in the Claire Sylvia case was her sudden craving for beer in front of the two reporters just a few short days after she received her new heart and lungs. It seemed to suggest somehow that in the early battle between acceptance and rejection her spirit was coming to terms with a whole new entity within her body. What about me?

Only a couple of odd things happened during my initial recovery, although at the time it was very easy to dismiss. The first was my request when I was asked if I would like anything to eat. It felt like a question that shouldn't need much thinking. I was tired, I felt very rough and I could hardly speak. The natural response would be the first thing that came into my mind, a favourite or common food item. My answer. "Rhubarb yoghurt please". Rhubarb? Yoghurt? Both in the same pot? I know me, I should be having brie, a nice cup of tea, maybe some monster munch, a Kit Kat and a four finger one too. But rhubarb yoghurt? Clearly that was wrong.

So was that my first sign? It would seem odd if it was. And also slightly annoying. Claire Sylvia got beer and fried chicken. I get rhubarb yoghurt.

The other strange event was the people that entered my room during my spell in intensive care. Most were professionals going about their business or family members taking their turns to keep my company. One person certainly was not meant to be there; mainly because he'd make so much noise he'd keep the whole hospital awake. I'd started hallucinating and my visions took the form of one Jimi Hendrix, and I have to say it was enjoyable. Jimi didn't really play that much for me, but he'd sit at the end of the bed, beside a cracking home made fire and just shoot the breeze. In many ways he seemed flattered to know me, as though I was the idol here. I'm not a fan of mind altering drugs generally, but at a time of significant pain, I certainly would recommend them. I loved the guitar and was a Hendrix fan, so at least this vision made sense to me, and I suspect had nothing to do with the new organ inside me.

Life remained a blur in those first couple of days, my memories limited to the odd moment of pain when drainage tubes and catheters had to be removed. It's odd how you don't notice these things attached to you; I certainly hadn't realised I had a catheter fitted. How I thought I was going to the toilet is anyone's guess. It wasn't until I found myself admiring a rather pleasant nurse that I realised there was something more going on down there. A pleasant thought soon turned into a shocking surprise.

If the addition of these various tubes had gone unnoticed, then removing them wasn't quite as stealthy as I would like. I have learned that when a nurse asks you to count down from three, she is generally going to pull out the offending item on two. There is a limited number of times that trick can work before someone just refuses to count. I am that man.

Before long I was back in the normal ward, with my own private room looking out onto Papworth Hospital's famous duck pond. My recovery was much the same as anyone else going through a form of open heart surgery. The big difference was getting used to the huge quantities of anti-rejection medicine I was taking, and just dealing with the psychological impacts of having a transplant.

The drugs very quickly made me feel sick, and indeed some of the liquids I was asked to drink were almost impossible to get past your nose, the smell was so disgusting. In fact for ages after, just smelling petrol at a petrol station would be enough to make me wretch, the smell reminded me of some of the substances I had to take.

Physically progress was swift; I was on an exercise bike within a few days, and walking a reasonable distance after just a couple of weeks. Mentally the challenge was only just beginning. I had already realised that what I was getting was not going to be a cure from the genetic disorder I had inherited, but more that I would be swapping one set of problems for another. More importantly there were very little guarantees about survival rates. My future was more uncertain than it had ever been, and there was also the small matter of knowing someone had died just for me to get this far.

Now I'm not really a crying type of person. Like most men I save my tearful moments for the things that really matter, like watching my football team win a trophy, but as I started to feel stronger emotional feelings that my body had suppressed when I was weaker started bubbling to the surface.

It was the usual morning routine on the ward and I had already eaten breakfast and managed to get myself washed and shaved, despite having to wheel a pole containing a few drips with me. I was now back on my bed, tired from the mornings exertions, and relaxing by listening to the radio on my Walkman. I'm not ashamed to admit that the music playing that morning caused me to cry uncontrollably. I'm not ashamed that it was the first moment that I'd thought about my donor and realised that another family was in pain. I'm not ashamed that it took a male nurse to comfort me and to help me gain my composure again. I am though, very ashamed to admit that it was Boyz II Men playing that morning and the track was "End of the Road". There I've said it.

I've often wondered what made me cry that morning. I've always just assumed that I finally had time to think what had happened to me, rather than have to fight some pain or force some medication down. It was going to come out at some point and that it came out to Boyz II Men was just a coincidence. I take a look through the lyrics for the first time, as I really can't remember the song that well.

Although we've come
To the end of the road
Still I can't let go
It's unnatural
You belong to me
I belong to you

Did my subconscious attach more meaning to those lyrics and set my train of thought immediately to my donor? Or was it something more? I doubt it, but if my donor ends up being a rhubarb yoghurt eating Boyz II Men fan, I'll certainly take it as 100% proof that cellular memory exists.

Reflections

"Most of all, my feelings are with those people waiting for donation whose lives depend upon having an organ through transplantation."

Mark Drakeford (the Welsh health minister after a vote was passed in favour of presumed consent in Wales)

Something has been bothering me since I came back from Paris, and a subsequent Twitter conversation has only added to my feelings of doubt.

It started with a comment about the change to presumed consent for organ donation that was passed by the Welsh Assembly. Presumed consent means that every individual will have presumed to have consented for their organs to be donated unless they opt out. This is a hugely positive change for the donation process and could hopefully help to save lives that might otherwise be lost on the transplant list.

Am I in favour of such a move? If it leads to more transplants then of course I am; anything that could have saved the life of my brother will always be welcomed by me. But today on Twitter, I just wanted to point out something about my donor that makes me feel very proud. My donor made the decision to pick up a donor card, to fill it in, to discuss his feelings with his family. It was a conscious decision, and that comforts me massively. I know it was something he felt was right to do.

The benefit of opting in is just that, you know that the donors are the ones that do have a real belief in what they are signing up for. What I would really like is for everyone to be educated so that enough people registered on the donor register without the need for presumed consent.

Sadly I know that will not happen, so presumed consent has to be the way forward.

With Twitters limitation of 140 characters, my comments may have come across as someone who thought the Welsh were wrong in their decision. I needed a minimum of 150 characters to explain myself. Maybe Twitter needs some kind of extension capability for those about to put their foot firmly in their mouth.

As the conversation rumbled on between a host of transplantees and donor family members another comment appeared that naturally took my eye.

This was a post that was attempting to educate readers to the common urban myths about transplantation, and this particular myth was that you don't take on the characteristics of the donor following transplant. Curious, I replied and suggested that whilst unlikely, some recipients had felt changes. Before too long I was in a short conversation about the subject and strangely for me I was falling on the side that was open to it. Clearly my investigations were having an effect on me.

What happened next though was something I really wanted to avoid. A mother of a donor joined the conversation. My heart jumped more than one beat as I tried my best to close the conversation down. It's not that I didn't want to discuss it, but how do you know how someone is really feeling over a medium such as social media. It's not the place to go over the psychological or physiological impacts of having a donor organ placed inside you so you may live. I was scared I would offend her, and it made me question this whole process. Should I carry on? What would the families make of my search for my donor? Maybe I shouldn't draw too many conclusions but just get to the end of the process quietly and see what it really reveals to me.

Of course much of my study is light hearted. It's hard to expect to understand the donor within by just making a trip up the Eiffel Tower, it's not intended to be scientific but just a search for myself. Hopefully on reading this people understand that. I'm not sure I did at the beginning myself.

So is there a type of transplant patient that would be particularly open to feeling the changes that cellular memory might bring? In Pearsall's research he suggested that about 1 in 10 patients have the kind of mind that can tap into their heart's energy and become sensitive to the other side of their being. Where that leaves the liver and kidney patients I'm not sure, but I'm guessing we can listen to those organs too. I know my brain listens very closely to one of my organs but not the one Pearsall was talking about.

Worrying that I won't be open to my heart's energy and "cardio-sensitive", I start to read through the key characteristics of someone able to get in touch with the other side of their being.

A feminine point of view - an early win, I made a heart shaped photo frame for my car called Tilly, last year. I rest my case. 1-0 Watson.

Open minded - an odd one as you would think Pearsall could do away with the other characteristics and just leave it as this. However as an open minded person I read on. 2-0 Watson.

Body aware - apparently this is being in control of your motions. I've been found naked on a friend's bathroom floor clearly not fully in control of my motions. 2-1 Watson.

Music lover - there isn't a person on this earth that wouldn't be impressed with my banjo skills and harmonica playing. 3-1 Watson. It's a good start.

Highly creative - many patients reported that they loved to read or write. I'm writing this, and you don't get much more creative than my own 6 track version of "Little Donkey". 4-1 Watson.

Environmentally sensitive - this seems more to do with remembering little details of places, rather than ensuring your loo paper is recycled. I do recycle, but my mind is a sieve. 4-2 Watson.

Good visualisation ability - surely that's the ability to see? I can see. I can also visualise me scoring the winning goal at Wembley. Possibly the greatest goal of the little known 1978 mini World Cup. 5-2 Watson.

Physic-sensitive - I'm going to lose my 'open minded' score in a minute. Supposedly being sensitive to things other people are not sensitive to. Does my allergy to peanuts count? 5-3 Watson.

Dependent - trusting and dependent on others. I trusted my brother and it cost me several injuries. I've learned my lesson and I'm more a loner. Think Benji the Littlest Hobo but with a drier nose and less problem solving skills. 5-4 Watson.

Compulsive - small repetitive type behaviour. We all have our compulsions, mine seems to be sitting in front of the football swearing loudly at Andy Townsend. Not sure it counts. 5-5 I'm slipping fast.

Unresolved grief - Ah. Pearsall describes a person with "a chronic, mildly depressive nature sometimes masked by self-deprecating humour". Who thought depression could put you back in the lead. Think I've answered his point. 6-5 Watson.

Animal loving - five cats, three dogs, a hamster with no fur and one eye, a ferret with a heart condition, a lost tortoise, a fish that made its way to my granddads cup of tea, several guinea pigs and two cows that went to slaughter. I've had them. They have all met their deaths. 6-6 Draw.

Climate sensitive - I don't talk to plants, I generally kill them through lack of love and attention. But Pearsall mentions allergies and I sneeze, itch and come out in hives watching the Sunday Gardening Show. 7-6 Watson.

Involved - in a large group I'm quick to want to get back to being by myself. Not so much a wallflower, more a great big prickly cactus enjoying the sun in its own piece of desert. Well an ex-partner said I was prickly anyway. I think that's what she said. 7-7 Draw.

Dreamer - are nightmares classed as dreams? I go to bed on a diet of blue cheese, Jack Daniels and the odd antihistamine and all that happens is I get attacked by Barny the flying spider. I'll wipe that smirk off his face one day. Not sure it's what we are looking for here. 7-8 Pearsall.

Sensual - hello ladies. Ah, this appears to be more about being gentle. See the previous "prickly" comment. I enjoy holding hands, but more of the good solid handshake type after another great badminton win. 7-9 Pearsall.

Ectomorphic - apparently slender, narrow faces, underweight with dark eyes. If I look at school photos of myself I look positively malnourished. Currently I am more slender with the gentle curve of an athlete's stomach. If you consider darts players athletes. I'm claiming this though. 8-9 Pearsall.

"Flow-er" more than "fighter" - I've only resorted to physical violence once. My brother was teasing me and I said I'd hit him with my guitar unless he stopped. He didn't. The guitar smashed over his head. I cried. With that bit of positive news the final score is a 9-9 draw!

So what does all this tell us? It reminds me that I probably need counselling more than I think I do, and that I should report my lack of control of my motions to the hospital. Maybe not.

It doesn't seem too bad. I'm not the type of person most in tune with my hearts energy and I can see that Claire Sylvia would have fitted the profile well. After all she was artistic, open minded and one who listened to her dreams. As much as I admire Sylvia for talking about the subject of transplants so openly, we are too dissimilar for me to really relate to the character traits she possessed pre-transplant. I need to relate to someone I would more naturally be drawn to. A hero.

Like most children of the 70's I lived for my action heroes, the kind of men that could take on a complete army themselves and come out fighting. Men that wouldn't flinch in the face of terrible nature. All these heroes were available to me in plastic form. My favourites were Action Man and the Six Million Dollar Man, who looking at now I kind of feel I've gone one step further by having my heart replaced. Take that Steve Austin. But my ultimate action figure was Evel Knievel, whose toy bikes used to race around the family hallways frightening the dog on regular occasions. I loved the sound as I wound the bike up to its maximum speed and then watched in awe as my little Evel careered into the skirting board.

The real Knievel was a daredevil stuntman who used to thrill audiences with his attempts at jumping buses on his variety of motorcycles, feats that left him with a world record amount of broken bones, estimated at 433 during his career.

Probably as a result of the many blood transfusions he received over the course of his life, Knievel contracted hepatitis C and after a long battle with the illness was finally given a liver transplant in 1999, following the death of a young motorcyclist.

This was more the kind of person I could look up to and believe in, but despite all the stories that surrounded Evel

Knievel's life, there was not much information to be discovered about his feelings following the life-saving operation. The only detail I could find was that he was "getting used to the medication", something even the ruthlessly tough Knievel found difficulty with.

Evel Knievel died on 30th November 2007 following another battle with diabetes and idiopathic pulmonary fibrosis. I suspect Knievel was unlikely to have felt any changes in his characteristics, he had probably already experienced much of life and it may have been hard to spot subtle changes when he had been so used to letting his body heal from so many injuries. If you are the type of person that breaks your pelvis in front of 90,000 people and still speak to the crowd afterwards, then you are unlikely to admit to feeling odd about liking a different food type all of a sudden.

As I read through the archives, another name began to crop up. This man was Bill Wohl, a former collegiate and professional athlete who had built up his own business in Scottsdale, Arizona. Bill's company worked at high profile events such as the Olympic Games and World Cups, but life was hectic and stressful.

In 1999 Wohl suffered what he initially thought was food positioning, but what turned out to be a major heart attack. Life was about to get very different and after major surgery Bill was still left with a heart functioning at only 15% of capacity.

At first Wohl was told he was too ill for transplant, something which confuses a lot of people who have never met anyone either waiting on the list or with a transplant. To be placed on the list for a transplant operation you need to be ill enough that there is no other option open apart from the transplant itself, yet your body must be strong enough to be able to cope with both the operation and subsequent recovery. As organs are in limited supply, it doesn't make sense to waste one on someone who is unlikely to make it through, no matter how horrible that decision may seem.

Fortunately for Wohl though, the improvements in medical science meant that a totally artificial heart was now available. Once placed in his body the mechanical device could pump blood round his body allowing him a small window to make improvements in his overall health.

On a video we can see Wohl working out with the artificial heart pumping blood beside him. Wohl looks plump of face and looks fitter than me on my good days, but as many patients know, looks can be deceptive and crucially time was running out. Finally after recovering enough to be accepted on the transplant list, Wohl got the gift of life with an operation on 22nd February 2000.

Wohl had previously been a hard working businessman who knew how to operate in a cut throat environment, yet after the operation he started to sense changes.

"Amidst all the challenges I faced with rehabilitation from my transplant, I was keenly aware that my values, feelings and life choices were mysteriously shifting. As miraculous and monumental as my heart transplant was, I just couldn't attribute the changes to that. I knew there was something very profound happening."

Like myself, Wohl also had a strange reaction to a piece of music he wouldn't have normally listened to, or had ever heard before. Whilst driving his car, Wohl was listening to a station he hadn't tuned into before when he heard a song by the British artist Sade. Immediately he broke down and cried, yet couldn't quite understand why the song had such an emotional effect on him.

Wohl's donor had been a young Hollywood stuntman named Michael Brady, who had performed hundreds of stunts without ever getting seriously injured. Sadly, Brady actually died preparing for a stunt, slipping from an extension ladder and suffering a fatal fall hitting his head on a river rock. Brady had always been a spiritual and caring man, looking to help those less fortunate than himself. He had only been in the fifth grade at school when he had written an essay saying that he wanted to be an organ donor. He was only 36 at the time of his death.

Nine months following his transplant Wohl had his first contact with his donor's family. They spoke, and afterwards he sent them a CD of Sade's songs explaining that it had moved him greatly, yet he was unsure as to why. He just wanted to share the lyrics with them.

"I spoke with Michael's brother Chris and he said that Sade was one of Brady's favourite artists."

Wohl seems someone I can relate to, especially given his experience with the music of Sade and his donor. It leaves me feeling more positive that my own emotional response to Boyz II Men could be something more than just the tears from someone who has just realised their life has been saved.

I look again through the list of characteristics that Pearsall says is typical of patients that are able to sense cellular memory, and I can't imagine them applying to a hard-nosed, athletic businessman. If Wohl can experience these types of changes then surely I can as well. As Lennon once sang "You may say I'm a dreamer, but I'm not the only one". My hope has returned.

Pearsall does offer some advice to getting more in touch with a donated organ. It seems that those patients who had deliberately tried to sense changes in their character had struggled or became frustrated in their attempts. Most of the changes, like Sylvia's sudden admission of a liking for beer, or Wohl's breaking down at the lyrics of Sade, had just come through quite naturally and without forethought. If my experiments are going to be a true test, I need to try and let the experiences just happen. In Paris I had tried to feel my donor's spirit as I made my way to the top of the Tower, but maybe that had been a mistake.

The stories of Wohl and Evel Kenievel had reminded me that as a child I always wanted to be the tough guy. I never was, but there was always the little daredevil in me, the little Kenievel, I just had to find it again.

Test 2 - The Slope

"I was more nervous to meet them than I was for my Olympic race. I mean, how do you thank somebody for saving your life at the same time they just endured a horrible family tragedy?"

Chris Klug (professional alpine snowboarder and liver transplantee who won a bronze medal in the Parallel Giant Slalom at the 2002 Winter Olympics)

Most people with an older brother will know that their love is usually demonstrated through means that will generally cause pain, embarrassment and feelings of defeat. My brother, Adrian, was no different.

I'm not quite sure how much he felt that he should protect me. I was always the sickly child, wheezing from asthma, throwing up from an allergic reaction to nuts or having my odd epileptic fit. Adrian on the other hand was big, strong and able to puff a few illegal cigarettes without so much of a sore throat. Any gestures of care towards me were no doubt designed to push me harder and toughen me up. He was kind like that and so we came to "the slope".

Norfolk isn't a place renowned for its undulating hillside or mountainous scenery. The best views you can get of our countryside are generally formed by climbing some kind of tree tower or out from the top of an old council building. We have an extremely flat county and one of which we are proud.

But for any Norfolk boy, the smallest little mound is going to have a magnetic pull to it. Many of my childhood photos show me atop a small heap of dirt, proudly looking as though I have claimed Everest. A hill was to be climbed, to be explored, and to claim with a flag, just that in this county that generally took sixty seconds to do.

Despite the limited options, one slope always drew me and Adrian to it, being situated just a few strides away from our home. It was a humble street, just a handful of houses long, but with the steepest descent we'd ever laid our eyes on. With most roads you'll see a sign with the gradient of the climb on it. No such need. This was unclassified, mainly as I suspect it was too gentle a hill, and secondly because Norfolk Council didn't realise those types of signs existed.

From the top of this vista the eye could see, well pretty much as far as the bottom of the slope. Even so, on a regular basis we might cycle up and down it, or just marvel at its sheer un-flatness. One day though, Adrian had a better idea. We had just built a small kart, made of wood with some child size bicycle wheels attached. This was a typical kart of the time, all homemade, string for steering and of course no need for brakes. Who wants to stop when you're ten years old?

Sensibly, Adrian was aware of the lack of brakes and also the height of the hill, and putting two and two together had decided the first run should be mine. Always kind. Always thinking. I too, had worked this concept out as well, and naturally questioned the decision to proceed down the slope without any form of stopping. Even at ten, I knew I wasn't going anywhere if safety wasn't an option, and who do you look to for that advice than your big brother.

"Don't worry, it'll be Ok", Adrian advised. "I'll go to the bottom and put my leg out to stop you".

How could that fail I thought? Adrian knows what he's doing, and better his leg than mine. The fool, that's surely going to hurt? A chance to pay him back for all the pain he has caused me. Win-win.

So Adrian went down the slope. I climbed into my kart, eagerly waiting as Adrian manoeuvred into position. The leg came out and the signal was set. I lifted my feet from the floor, tucked them into the box and immediately it felt like a speed that only a chosen few daredevils had reached. Half way down and this was scary, faster than I'd anticipated, maybe faster than Adrian anticipated. But as I stared intently at my safety buffer of my brother's leg, something suddenly jolted my mind. His leg wasn't there! He'd pulled it back and now was smiling gleefully as I raced down a hill that at its bottom was traversed by another street. His smile showed a look of joy at the many possible outcomes that could come from this trick, all of them ending in my discomfort.

Within seconds I raced past where Adrian was sitting, my safety net had gone and all that could stop me now was a collision with something solid. Luckily that something was not a car coming along the street at the bottom of the slope, but it was a stationery car parked in a resident's garage, and that was being worked on too. I didn't have enough time to shout out in pain as I hot-footed it away with the kart before even more trouble befell me.

And so begun my hatred for any downhill activity, and also my lack of trust for anything my brother ever said.

Today is very similar day, or at least from memory it feels similar in that it's a beautiful hot summer's day, the type of day that has newspapers telling you how much hotter we are than the Mediterranean. A perfect day to get back to the slope then, to see what's different and if my donor heart feels more comfortable with this "extreme" sport environment than me. But surely I'd look silly in a kart on a housing estate at my age, so instead I've made my way to a bigger slope, bigger than any hill Norfolk has to offer. I'm at the Milton Keynes Snodome.

I've come here with my good friend Sarah, both to try out Snowboarding for the first time and also to do some sledging, which to me felt the closest activity I could find without actually looking like an overgrown child. Even so, on the drive up there my mind and stomach have been feeling a mixture of excitement and nerves. I'm loving the idea of snow and looking cool, I'm less enjoying the thought of me coming home on crutches, something my brother would surely have liked.

As we pull up in the car the Snodome looks grey and bland, but the size of it is larger than we both expected. Nervousness appears and despite the heat I feel a shiver go down my back. Adrian at least only put me at the top of a small incline; this looks much more daunting and would surely take more than a leg to stop anyone coming down from this height.

We find a space in the car park, jump out and pull our bags from the boot of my car. It's been hard to know what to pack, after all we are in the middle of a heat wave and we are about to enter a freezing cold and snowy environment. I don't go out in the snow these days. Well not if I can help it at least. Snow to me means delays, traffic, danger and endless stories about a lack of salt on the local news. Gone are the days when it was a source of excitement and pleasure.

Once inside we pick up our tickets for the sledging. When I booked I thought this would be the closest thing to my old kart, and a good introduction before we got down to the business of trying to look cool on a snowboard. We are directed through to the changing rooms, where the heat is still as hot and muggy as it was outside. It feels a tad strange to be putting on more layers. From my bag I pull a base layer, a t-shirt, grey combat trousers and an orange waterproof jacket. Most people look fairly hip when snowboarding, I on the other hand worry I look like a road sweeper heading out for an annual convention. No one else is in the changing room as I look around for a bit of reassurance, so I am forced into stepping outside and hoping I don't stand out too much as a real amateur, which of course is what I am.

Sarah has already changed and from her expression I can tell she feels as inappropriately dressed as I do. She has gone for a hoody and some tracksuit bottoms, a slightly better look but one that worries her into thinking she is going to be frozen over the next few hours. We walk to the desk, smile, and ask where we go for the sledging. The guy at the desk looks neither amused nor concerned about our appearance and tells us to wait over by the seats and someone will take us through in a moment. I feel slightly concerned that there is no-one else here. Perhaps everyone is at the beach, maybe I should be.

We are taken to what at first appears to be a giant meat packing refrigerator. It has those same plastic strips covering the entrance, the sort of thing you see in the movies, where you go through inevitability leads to a dead body. I really hope there are no dead bodies. Fortunately as I step through it reveals the slope, which has lost a lot of its daunting height. It's still large, but the interior seems much less in scale than the exterior, and the slope we are heading to goes only half way up. This should be easy I think to myself.

We are in a small group, there is me and Sarah and then two small children with their parents. The children are far too excited about the snow and this certainly looks a first too for the parents, as the father is dressed in the thickest snow jacket I've ever seen, his glasses just peering out through the hood.

We all pick up our trays. These are just round discs that remind me of the old tea trays I used to use, except slightly more tasteful. As we climb the hill I watch the children, looking to see which one is the more dominant sibling, the one with the confidence and cheek my brother used to show. Sadly they both seem quite similar in age and as they race up the hill, they just shriek at each other and help as they, in turn, fall over in their excitement. We watch as both of them place their trays down. Unlike with Adrian and me, they both look to each other for reassurance and then proceed to head down the slope. Slow at first they soon start spinning round in circles, until one of the brothers catches a lump in the snow and tumbles over. He lays there for a while. Maybe this could have a danger element to it? A moment passes, we all look on in concern, but suddenly there is movement and he is back on his tray and slowly edging to the bottom.

Now it's our turn. I place the tray down on the snow. I try and imagine Adrian at the bottom of the slope willing me to come down, his leg stretched out in front of him like some reassuring bumper. I place myself on the tray, and stare hard at the vision I've created. I can almost see Adrian now, and I can feel the trust I always placed in him in these moments. I push off and my weight makes it a slower start than I'd hoped for, but within a few seconds the lack of friction sees me picking up the pace rapidly. Suddenly I'm twisted backwards, and I'm going very fast but the wrong way round. I've lost Adrian, but I'm smiling, and although I can't see where I'm going the fun of it all makes it hard not to relax. As I come to the bottom, no leg stops me, no road awaits me, but I do come off the tray and end up face first in the snow. Brilliant.

We carry on going up and down the slope using a variety of sledges, some of which are the more traditional type. I test the true nature of the snow by tipping some down Sarah's back. It's definitely the real stuff, the noise she makes confirms it.

Just as I'm feeling more relaxed the father of the children comes hurtling past us at a speed that suggests he is very much out of control. He's nearing the bottom of the slope, and just like the young me, he hasn't got anyone to stop him.

The panic suggests that he is now awaiting some pain, and the only thing that can stop him now is something solid. Sure enough he misses the barrier that runs across the bottom of the slope and proceeds to go right through some orange mesh netting, taking two support poles along with him as he finally comes to a shuddering stop. He looks like a fly caught in a spider's web. A fly with very steamed up glasses and a snow jacket that has tried to escape over his head. Sarah chuckles. When Sarah chuckles it means one of two things, either something was funny, or she is nervous. I suspect it's both.

The session ends and we have some time before the real reason for our trip begins, our first snowboarding lessons. Feeling cold we head back into the warmth and get a drink to replenish some energy. Sarah has a very cultured coffee, I on the other hand have a slush puppy. Seems I can't get enough of the cold right now.

It certainly reminds me of my childhood, sitting in my cold damp clothes that, whilst slowly warming, do not actually get any drier. I know as a child heading back to the snow already damp meant you pretty soon became frozen. Sitting like this it's hard to remember that it's currently 28 degrees outside.

Rested we head back over to the desk where all the equipment is stored and hand over our tickets for the lesson. We are the first here and we are immediately handed some boots and a snowboard each. We sit ourselves down and proceed to pull the boots onto our feet.

I suspect seasoned snowboarders know how to get these things on easily, but I've only managed to get one foot half way in and can't seem to pull it on any further or even pull it off again. Finally I try one last big effort, my head between my knees as I heave and grunt. Sarah is in a fit of giggles. She can't stop laughing yet I'm flushed red, not wanting to give in at this stage. Suddenly the boot gives, my foot slips, and I return to an upright position whilst Sarah collapses on the bench crying in laughter. I picked the right person for support today it would appear.

Booted up we then move to the helmets. We pick the bright yellow ones that are sized in small, medium and large. I put a small on my head, and Sarah's giggles tell me I've picked the wrong one. Medium goes snugly on and feels like it may offer some protection. I suggest we test them out, so we take a pace back, and then step forward bashing our heads against each other. Luckily no one witnesses this ceremony, and the helmets do their job.

We are now joined by our other first time snowboarders, who are two young girls, both appear as nervously excited as we are. This feels like a good sign. I'm not at my most confident when in a group of physically fit males. My strength following transplant makes me feel slightly inadequate when in that type of group. Hopefully I won't let anyone down. My thoughts have drifted naturally to my donor, and there is a feeling that I should this, for them. I don't really know if it's what they would enjoy, I just know I've been given an opportunity to enjoy this new experience and I don't want to be held back by fear.

As we go back out to the slope, we get a few basic instructions about how to attach ourselves to the board, and how our weight and body positioning will control what the board does. All seems very straightforward at this stage. The instructor then points up the slope, up past the slope we used earlier, past a little ledge in the distance and right up to the top of the cold, grey building. Hmm, I'm not so sure now.

To make this easier, he states we will be coming down backwards, using the toe edge of the board to control our descent. He did say "backwards" didn't he? This is the first lesson right? Bugger.

We make our way onto the little escalator taking us up the slope, clutching onto our snowboards like some kind of comfort blanket. It takes an age to reach the top and from here the slope looks bigger and more severe than before. One word is still running around my head. "Backwards".

We are told to spread out in a line, and then shown how best to proceed to the edge of the slope. I'm trying to listen to the instructions, they generally consist of some sort of rolling over, but my head can only hear my brother's instructions to me. That I'd be safe. That he'd stop me. The instructor exudes the same confidence, and that it's easy and safe. "Lying bastard" I think.

Having not paid attention I'm now feeling extra nervous as one by one we get ready for our first attempts. I would assume any alpha male would immediately step forward and be the first to show how it's done. Obviously I'm no alpha male, and I feel certainty in my mind that my donor isn't either. I want to be, I am just not built that way, and even my change of heart has not altered that.

I watch as the two other girls from the group edge forward. The first makes slow but steady progress down the snow. Hmm. The next takes a little longer, and just as she gets to her feet, she is over again, bottom in the air, hands planted in the snow on front of her. Horrible I know, but I'm happy. I may fail here, but I'll be failing in company. I like that.

Sarah is next and I certainly don't want her to fail. Well maybe a little bit. Maybe like Eddie "The Eagle" Edwards. A heroic failing. She shuffles back over the edge, balances, and starts slowly sliding her way down. She looks good. Wobbly maybe, but good. She starts to catch up to the other girls, and nicely for me takes one of them out by colliding into her just as she'd found her footing. This is going well!

Just as my confidence soars the instructor tries to ruin it. "You're the only man today. Chance to show them how it's done" he says.

This doesn't feel the time to get into a debate about sexism, and his good intentions are to make me feel relaxed before I start. However the pressure now feels back on me.

As I start to shuffle nearer towards the edge my legs start to wobble a little, I stretch myself gently upright and without thinking I start to slide very slowly down the slope. This feels easier than I imagine, but my heart is racing so fast it's hard to keep control of my breathing. I try singing to myself. Out loud. Luckily it's not the Boyz II Men tune from my recovery days, but just some random words being shouted out to a made up backing track. I certainly look a little odd, but I don't think anyone notices, and before too long I find myself coming to a standstill with the slope stretching out ahead of me. I've done it! I've completed my first snowboard run, and I didn't even need my brother's legs to stop me.

I congratulate one of the girls who has made it down with me and try to look like the confident sort of guy that does this all the time. I don't think she is fooled, but we both look up to see Sarah making her way down. Still giggling, still hard to tell what that giggle means.

We all head back up the escalator, ready for our next runs. My confidence is helped further by the final member of our quarter still being unable to stand up. I hate myself for enjoying the fact I'm not the worst snowboarder in the world, but the feeling of achievement leaves me wanting more.

We continue the process of going backwards down the slope for a good forty-five minutes. There doesn't appear to be any great instructions, but the freedom to just keep trying reminds me of how I learnt best as a child. Get up, fall down, get up again. I like this.

Is it my childhood I'm remembering here, or is there an element of enjoyment coming from within that has something more to do with the transplanted me. I've tried not thinking of my donor, but every now and then it slips through. The one thing I do know is that I'm having a great time. My confidence is growing with each descent, and I'm hoping the session doesn't end.

We come to the last few minutes and we've been instructed to try going side to side. Most of the session I've been doing that even though I haven't intended to, so this seems an easy step to make.

Once again I'm the last to set off, and already there doesn't seem a set path that anyone is following. Sarah has made it a quarter of the way down but is on the floor trying to get her snowboard untangled. As I set off I seem to be a good distance from anyone else, but as I shift my weight and start to move myself from one side of the slope to the other, my speed picks up quickly.

Suddenly I'm heading towards Sarah's tangled legs, I'm moving at pace and unable to really change my course. The vision of Adrian's legs is flashing through my mind, and I feel just as out of control as I did then. Sarah can see me coming, but unlike Adrian, she doesn't pull away, more through the weight of the snowboard than any concern for slowing me down. We collide. Both of us are now in a heap in the snow, but unlike my childhood days, this feels an enjoyable part of the experience. We get up, dust the snow off and happily finish the session.

Snowboarding has brought out the child in me again, and maybe that just says this is something I always enjoyed doing. It's just that as an adult I've forgotten to try the things I did before. My donor may not feel part of this adventure, but it was him that got me here today, and for that I'm grateful. I will return.

The Ten Year Letter

"It is our experience that many patients have asked about their donor and many have wanted to say 'thank you' to the family of their donor. It has been shown that donor families react very positively on receiving such letters."

Papworth Hospital "Writing to your donor's family – A patients guide"

"Thank you for your letter, which we appreciate was difficult for you to write. The family are pleased to hear you are doing so well. It was our son's wish and we do not believe anyone should go against a person's wishes.

"We wish you and your family the very best for the future and once again appreciate the effort you made to write to us."

Sixty-six short words, but unless you are a recipient of a donor organ it's hard to convey what that little communication means to me. Without context it could read like a response to a job application, but let me take you through everything that I saw when I opened that card, almost ten years ago.

They got my letter, they actually have read my words. Just to know I've finally told someone how grateful I am, and that it's been received is like a bombshell to me. Amazing.

Then there's the "thank you". It's a sign they are pleased and thankful to hear from me. Imagine being told you have a letter from someone who has had a loved one's organs transplanted into them. They might not want to know, but I have a "thank you".

There's an understanding of how much of a painful process it was for me to write. I sense it's been difficult for them to receive my words too, but maybe they have been waiting years for this moment. I'm glad they know it hasn't been easy.

They are pleased I'm "doing so well". I spend my life trying to live up to this superhuman hero whose heart has saved my life. To hear those words makes me feel like my donor family are a little proud of me. Maybe that's too strong, but it's a big thing for me.

"It was our son's wish". His wish. His decision. He'd thought about it. He'd registered and talked it through with his family. I will always be eternally grateful for that. It's an act of such kindness and he probably never realised the impact that decision would make. He let me live. If you ever wanted a reason to join the donor register, that's it.

The next part of that line is more difficult. I've read it many times and I sense it was a decision that the family were not entirely comfortable with. Who can know what a family goes through in such fraught, emotional times? I couldn't think after Adrian died. They had to make a decision; maybe they felt they wanted to do it differently, but they stuck to their son's wishes. That's an amazing family. They did what he had asked, and I think that just shows the love they must have had for him.

They want me to go on being happy, and I'm thankful for those words. I've carried enormous guilt around with me.

Nothing I can do seems to stand up to the kindness of my donor. When I'm annoyed I feel I'm wasting the gift; when I'm happy I feel bad for just smiling. Maybe I can let that go a little? Maybe.

Finally they remind me of the difficulty in writing, and they've made the point twice. They waited a long time to hear from me. So long it made me feel sick. I worried that they would think I didn't care at all. At least they accept why. They know how hard this was.

Sixty-six words. No more, no less, but it says so much more.

As transplantees we all have the opportunity to write to our donor families, via a process the hospitals co-ordinate to ensure patient and donor confidentiality. I have no names, or address to go by. My letter had been an emotionally draining experience to write, and it had taken me ten years to do it. Ten years of juggling words around in my head. Ten years of ripping up bits of paper. Ten years of getting it wrong. Ten, long years full of guilt and shame.

So why did it take so long? Partly it's probably the lack of "Thanks for my organ" cards available in the shops. Ah, there it is again. Humour as a defence mechanism as I know there really isn't an excuse.

Initially, in those first few months, my donor was always a fleeting presence in my mind. I was dealing with rejection, changes in medication, blood transfusions and pipes up the majority of cavities you can find in your body. When I did have the energy to sense my donor it was too painful. The guilt was strong, I'd cry, my chest would hurt and it felt like my heart was beating so hard it was trying to make a break for it.

Six months in and I was back at work, tired and trying to get back to as normal a life as possible. My life became just a mix of work and sleep, lots of sleep. "Maybe tomorrow", I thought to myself, "maybe tomorrow, I'll think it through and find the words". Tomorrow never came.

Health began to return, but so did the desire to live faster, before the inevitable dying younger, and as such my relationship began to unravel. My life expectancy was never far from my mind, and now I also had lost my relationship and house through my own desire to live life day by day. I could write, but some days I just felt bitter. I'd been given an extension to my young life, I hadn't won the lottery. Those letters were short, looked ungrateful and quickly found their way to the bin.

A new relationship arrived as my head found a better place, but other events conspired to make my life tough. My health took a battering and suddenly it was all about staying well rather than writing letters. I wanted to be happy and healthy, but it always felt like a seesaw. I could be happy but not healthy, healthy but not happy. Not both. I'll write when I have both.

Next were thoughts of children. My friends were now building families, and as someone in their late twenties you start making decisions about the future. I was fearful, after all Adrian had died from this strange illness and it had affected me too. What did it all mean? When I was on the transplant list I'd been advised to freeze some of my semen, little swimmers frozen in time for use another day, mainly because the doctors were unsure of the drugs' effects on fertility. I stored two years worth inside a month, more tiring than impressive and without a magazine in sight. Sometimes the private medical practices don't live up to the good old NHS. But then again, what use was it? Wouldn't I be passing on this illness?

Genetic counselling was arranged. I've had quite a bit of counselling in my time, and this was a bit different. No discussion about how I felt about my genes, no trying to communicate with them in a clearer way, no reconciliation process, just blood tests, check-ups and trying to go as far through my family history as possible. At the end of a long process, I was told what I already knew. It was 50/50. I might pass it on, I might not. We'd only really know when the illness presented itself in any child. Russian roulette with sperm.

It's tricky for some people to understand. You were dying, but now you've had the miracle of a transplant and you're living. Hurray, life's amazing isn't it? Well yes it is, but at times, thinking of Adrian, going through yet another procedure, the survival rates running round your head and the decisions over children and the future, it was easy to feel bitter occasionally. Not the positive, happy, sugar-coated words that fall out of magazines about surviving health scares, but real emotions that runs deep within.

With those feelings bubbling to the surface sometimes, they inevitably seemed to appear on the page with any words I wrote. I may have jotted down "I'm loving life" on the paper, but that felt hollow and untrue. If I could see it, so would my donor family, "ungrateful bastard" was my imagined response. I didn't want that. I was utterly grateful. It was just that it was more difficult and complex than that.

Before too long, over 9 years had already passed and my donor family hadn't heard a peep from me. It was gnawing away at me and the pressure was growing, but after all this time would the hospital still hold any records?

First of all I just wanted to get the letter done. I'd tried and failed so many times, I didn't want to give anyone false hope about what I might do. I was also struggling with my own mortality, and I knew I still wasn't in the best position to write something that felt positive enough.

Why would anyone struggle so badly, so long after their initial transplant? Surely after a period of time you just settle into a normal life? I expect a lot of transplant patients do, but for me the statistics I'd been provided at my assessment were like little maggots eating away at the apple of my brain. They told me about how long I would live without a transplant, how many died during the operation, first year survival rates and a percentage of patients that die annually thereafter. They told me that only 50% survived 10 years, and that's where the statistics stopped.

As I moved through that first decade I heard of fellow patients I had known that had passed away, and I saw those patients who celebrated their tenth anniversary like they'd reached the biggest milestone in their life. But what went after it? No one had mentioned 20 or 30 year survival rates, it seemed to me like a cliff edge at the end of a long walk. You made your way down the winding path, tired but in the sunshine, made it to the cliff, wondered at the view and then..

My head was a swirl of emotions, I missed Adrian but I felt I hadn't really wanted to think about him for so long I'd forgotten who he was. I wanted my donor family to know I hadn't forgotten them either, but time was running out. There wasn't long to go before I was at that cliff edge. I needed to do something now before the inevitable fall.

I was at a major crossroads in my life again, another relationship at sink or swim stage. I needed to swim, and like any good patient I went to my GP for some armbands. Counselling was quickly arranged, and luckily for me we quickly built up a respect for each other. It felt like the right moment. An opportunity.

We worked through a lot of my feelings over the past 10 years. We walked through Adrian's death, holding his hand, the moment he reminded me of the cruel joke I'd made at his expense when he was first ill. As a younger brother opportunities for revenge were rare. This moment turned out to be the wrong time for it, but he comforted me in his darkest hours. We talked through my own operation and all that came after it. I was surprised how clear it was, how much I could connect with those hard times. Adrian felt closer and so did my donor. Pain didn't disappear at all, but love was allowed in, and that's all it needed.

I started to write out my feelings. Notes came and went, but it started to make more sense. There was gratitude, appreciation for what had been done for me, and I was able to sound happy with my life despite its turmoil. Life is life after all.

I shared my written thoughts first with my counsellor. Normally I had been the one crying, but as I read through my words it was impossible for any tears to be held back by either of us. I'd hit the mark. I was ready to send it off.

Even now, it makes me cry thinking about getting that letter out. A chance to connect. To say thank you. An immense burden of 10 years was starting to lift.

I can't remember how long it took to get a response, and whilst I wanted one, the important thing was just that I had written my letter. Even if the family didn't want it, at least they would know I had tried and that I cared. Life went on, and in keeping with the previous ten years it carried on in a chaotic manner, seeing long term goals pulled apart by moments of short term foolishness.

We should all feel like we are on a marathon, hopefully not hampered by wearing a huge elephant costume for added fun. We know the rough length of the marathon, and we know we need to save energy to get to the finish line. We don't rush, we enjoy the first 10-15 miles when we feel strongest and then push through the last 10, hearing the cheering crowds and enjoying the noise of the band. If you are lucky you may get a medal at the end of it.

In my life it feels like I know there is a marathon ahead of me, but I'm being chased by a lion the whole way. No point preserving energy, just run as fast as you can and hope not to get eaten, and all the while knowing in my head I'll never outrun the lion for 26 miles. It's going to get me, just a question of when. It doesn't make for a relaxing race, and the whole thing is full of fear and anxiety.

So now time has passed. I'm still being chased, but I've outrun the lion for more miles than I ever thought possible. But I'm exhausted. I'm not even half way through the marathon yet I have used all my reserves up. Someone needs to throw me a very large energy drink.

20 years is on the horizon and I feel the need to write again to my donor family. The pressure isn't anything like it was before, I doubt they are waiting or expecting anything from me now. They may have a lot more closure with their loss, and of course I wouldn't want to stir anything up again. But, I want to know. I want to know who this person is.

My hospital has confirmed they still hold records for my donor family, so there is no reason for me not to write. And I will. That ten year letter needed to express gratitude about the decisions both my donor and the family had to make in order for me to live. It was a thank you of epic proportions. This letter doesn't need to do that, it just needs to tell them about all the things I've achieved in life. Despite the frantic nature of my marathon, I've still helped people along the way, and that's all they need to know.

Life can be hard, frightening, exhausting and laden with anxious fears, but it is always cherished.

Now where is that damn medal?

The Birthday

"All participants were suffering end-stage heart failure at the time they were told that transplantation was the only option. For some it was the end of uncertainty and a hope; for others, feelings of insecurity and fear. All were aware that it would not be a choice, but the only chance of life."

"Experiencing heart transplantation: the patients' perspective" - a study by Noedir Antonio Groppo Stolf and Maria Lucia Araújo Sadala

The sound of jet planes booms overhead, breaking the peace and tranquillity of the Norfolk coastline. The sky is pure blue, the sea gently breaking across the pebble beach. It's my birthday. I'm 43 and I've taken the chance to find a little peaceful space for myself and unwind my busy head.

Ever since I started looking into cellular memory a number of things have happened that have left me unsettled. Unsure of my place in the world and uncomfortable with where I might be heading. I've started talking to many more transplantees, sometimes offering words of encouragement as they start their own journey, other times just listening, and hopefully reassuring those going through some of the anxieties we all face. After 19 long years, just the length of my survival makes me something of a reluctant role model.

I've spoken to some families, who have had to go through the trauma of donating loved one's organs. I've been amazed at their courage but more, their willingness to take the battle of organ donation wider, to be a voice for those still waiting on the list. Their loss is huge, their gift greater still.

I've started thinking about my own donor, more and more thoughts about him have filled my head. Of course that's the whole point of this book, but I didn't expect the range of emotions it has started to put me through, or the increased drive to be seen as fulfilling the life they left behind and gifted to me.

The trip to Paris and my snowboarding experiences have literally been just the tip of the iceberg. It's felt like my donor has been an increasingly close presence, and I find myself trying to understand my emotions in a multitude of different layers. Everything I do has to be understood in the context of my transplant and that has become increasingly traumatic, despite the enjoyment those events have given me.

I've thought about charities, starting them and promoting the thanks I feel to a wider audience. I've thought about how I could best fulfil my obligations to my donor before it's too late. I've become increasingly aware of my mortality, and this from someone whose mortality has always been front of mind.

I'm a man in the midst of a mid-life crisis. Coincidently I already own a small sports car, my partner is in her twenties and recently I nearly got myself stuck in a children's helicopter ride, the type you see outside supermarkets. I've not got much room to go further into this crisis apart from owning a pair of leather trousers. I've looked in all the stores. They are very hard to find. Maybe H&M should have a mid-life crisis range.

In short, the whole process of writing the book is having a traumatic effect on my life. It's already begun to have a destabilising effect on my relationship, like all the relationships that have fallen beside the wayside previously. Transplantation isn't for the faint-hearted. Admittedly, you may get to swap your faint heart for a much more robust one, but the effect is still the same. You have to be tough emotionally, and that's something I'm not.

Doctors are very clear, prior to going on the waiting list, about the risks and complications from being a transplantee, for instance the amount of people that just die waiting. Those that don't make it through the difficult operation itself. The fact that transplantation is not a cure, it's a life full of medication, fear of rejection and an organ with a limited shelf life as the body's limited immune system and the toll all the medication takes. You go into it fully accepting that this is an extension to your life, not a bright sunset of which to ride into.

When I had my transplant, my hope was for five more years, based on the figures at the time and the relative expectations other patients seemed to have. When I came up to ten years of survival I panicked. I thought it was coming to an end. No one had spoken about what came after and all I could see was the darkness of what lay ahead. I needed to blot it out, drink, go out, live life at 150 miles an hour until the collision came. It never came, but in its imagined wake, came a broken relationship, loss of my home and the need to rebuild yet again.

That same fear is enveloping me now. I'm heading towards my twentieth anniversary, something I never imagined would happen even in my most optimistic moments. I'm spinning around frantically trying to leave my legacy to the world, trying to get as fit as I can to stave off the inevitable, and my relationship is once again struggling too. I recognise the signs this time, but seem unable to rectify the situation. Luckily Jen is very understanding, but she has no clear direction of how best to help me.

The clouds appear to have closed out the blue sky above me now, both metaphorically and literally. Families sit and quietly chat, unperturbed by the change in weather. Most of the small groups here are parents or grandparents with their children and grandchildren. Life seems quite easy and simple by comparison, although the small cries from one small child suggest some basic needs are not being met.

I sit alone. 43 and surrounded by my chair, rug, empty ginger beer can and lunch box. It sounds like something from the Famous Five, except rather more lonely.

Yesterday I opened a birthday card from my mother. The front of the card was full of words displaying various positive characteristics. "You're generous" read one, "you're kind" read another. It seemed to be missing some of my other traits such as "you're very difficult to live with", "you break wind".

What was unnerving though was the printed inscription on the inside of the card. It read "it's genetic!" Clearly the purpose of this was to show that all those kind qualities the recipient has, are all handed down from the giver of the card. It's probably the narcissists' choice of card. My mother had missed this when buying it, and on opening the card the phrase became a much more macabre statement than I'm sure the makers intended. Your granddad is dead, your father is dead, your brother is dead but don't worry "it's genetic!". Happy birthday indeed.

Maybe I'm the only one that would see the statement that way. Maybe it's a reflection of my current state of mind, but as the clouds grow thicker I'm beginning to be more reflective on the failings in my life rather than the successes. Surely just being here 19 years following my donor's gift is a success itself? But if it's already a success, doesn't that mean failure is just around the corner? After all, if you spin a coin 15 times and it comes up heads, that's an amazing success, but you suspect 16 would be pushing your luck.

I pick up some stones from the beach and start to place them into two piles, one for success and one for failure. This seems like quite a good system as even I haven't had enough failings to run out of stones from this beach. I can also pick a stone the relative size of the success or failure thus providing a grading system. Maybe I've thought it through too much. Maybe that's what happens when you come to a beach alone.

Some ladies walk past inquisitively looking over to my rug and the few stones I'm collecting. They look bemused, as though they have come across a strange loner collecting rocks. I add another stone to the "failure" pile.

Successes soon stack up and I ensure I pick some hefty stones for my relative kindness, my volunteering, the fundraising I do and the time I give to helping friends. Smaller stones go to my ability in attracting kind ladies, my humour (though absent here), my patience, the ability to find decent bed and breakfasts, and being able to sleep the moment I hit the pillow.

Failures are defined by my lack of stability in relationships. I can't find a stone quite big enough, so plump for two medium ones. I imagine previous partners probably wanting to add a few stones themselves so put on another one just for luck. My inability to cope well with my transplant, my fear of pain of any sort and my nature of pushing away those who wish to get closer to me. This includes partners, friends with children and my limited amount of relatives. I still can't wee straight after 43 years and that surely deserves a pebble or two.

After a good while, I stop. The two mounds are both of fairly equal size. I have my faults, but obviously they are offset by my good points. Maybe that's good enough. After all, if you can accept your failings, then maybe you'll enjoy your successes.

The children and families have gone. A mist had started to descend but actually I now feel happier than when the sun was here.

We all have our failings, and in reality I'm just lucky that I have been given the opportunity by my donor to make the odd mess of things. I'm also sure that the people I do help in my life don't give a flying fig about any of my failings, they just see the good that is done. Equally those that I have hurt probably don't think any of my good work makes up for my shoddy behaviour. I'm no different to anyone else. I suspect if my donor was alive, they too would make the odd mistake. Sadly that chance has been taken from them.

The main purpose of this book was to find out who I really am. Everyone searches for their true identity and much of mine has been defined by my own health battles. My donor is clearly a huge part of the person I am. If someone had saved your life by pulling you from a burning car, wouldn't you want to know who they are? I'm the same with my donor, whilst also carrying part of their DNA around with me.

Maybe all the trauma, the sleepless nights I'm going through and the relationship difficulties are all part of that journey of finding the real me. Perhaps I need to go through these difficult moments in order to come out the other side with a truer perspective on the person I've become, and the donor that helped me live.

It's scary, and I can't hide away from my mortality either. That is also a part of who I am, just someone that has had to live with the knowledge that life can be taken away quite quickly. Lots of people live with that, and in a world perspective I have a lot more certainty about my life than most.

I'd wondered if I should stop writing, stop the experiment and go back to a life where I avoided talking to others in my situation. I've thought back about the words of encouragement that Amara had about finding peace. This whole journey is going to be a lot more difficult than I ever thought it would be. It's going to open up a lot of wounds but also a lot of real benefits and new friends.

I'd hoped the journey would be more of a celebration, a happy year spent finding the fun in life again and living a life I thought my donor would have loved. I don't want it to end up creating misery and pain, so I need to go back to the enjoyment of the Eiffel Tower and the Snodome. Enjoy life and just live it.

I head home, the clouds disappearing behind me, and I look forward to the chapters yet to be written.

Test 3 - Fiddle This

"I'm real sad for the guy who died and gave me his heart, but I really have trouble with the fact that he was black. I used to hate classical music, but now I love it. So I know it's not my new heart, because a black guy from the 'hood wouldn't be into that."

Case number 4 from research by Paul Pearsall. The 17 year old donor was walking to his violin class when he was killed in a drive-by shooting.

It's 11:17 in East London and the sign on the overground shows the next train to Stratford will be in 32 minutes time. Judging by Google that means I'm going to miss the last Central Line tube to Epping, where my car is sitting, waiting to carry me home.

I'm wondering why I'm in this predicament, and looking back at the event that took me out late on a Sunday night. I've been to Café OTO in Dalston, to see a rather quiet yet eccentric American called Frank Fairfield. Fairfield is a Californian fiddle, banjo and guitar player who seems to have stepped right out from a different era. Despite his youth he takes on the appearance of an old time musician with granddad shirt, oversized tweed trousers and a moustache that's more overgrown than trimmed.

I've been trying not prejudge what my donor's musical tastes might have been, but tonight the notion of cellular memory has entered my mind. Fairfield is someone who I have seen once before, at a festival a couple of years ago, but as I sit watching the clock slowly click by, it strikes me that Fairfield's fiddle playing is quite a departure from the music I liked before my operation.

The majority of us will alter our taste in music as we get older, (although some people do seem to stick with the 80's in an unnerving haircut kind of way) but we are often influenced by the world around us, friends, radio or even the odd advert. I ask Sean, my long term friend and gig companion if he can remember who introduced Fairfield to who? At this stage of the night, I'll be lucky if Sean can remember what his last name is, as his eyes glaze and stare heavily at the empty tracks in front of us.

"You told me I would like him, so I then went and bought his albums. It's why we went to that first End of the Road festival."

So this was my choice, and I know how much I hated playing both the violin and the viola as a child. I played in a school orchestra that included talented youngsters that would go on to compete in the BBC's "Young Musician of the Year" programme (maybe that's another show due a celebrity spin off). I was very much the child that destroyed the harmonious sound of our classical music with my ability to only find the wrong note at the wrong time. I was awful, although I do have a grade 2.

So after my traumatic experience with violins, what am I doing enjoying a night with a fiddle player in the surrounds of a small café, with the usual chalkboard menus and extortionate beer prices. Maybe, down the years, my donor heart has been pushing me back in this direction. Maybe I like the violin more than I think, and maybe I'm more talented than a Grade 2. As the train finally pulls in, I'm ready to resurrect my musical career.

There seems to have been a number of cases where transplant patients have gained different musical experiences. For some it can be finding a musical talent they didn't know existed and others it can just be a simple but dramatic change in musical taste.

The first case mentioned on Paul Pearsall's report into the changes of heart transplant recipients is about an 18 year old girl diagnosed with endocarditis and heart failure. Her donor had been an 18 year old boy with a love for writing his own poetry. The transplant had a profound effect on the young recipient, especially after hearing some of the songs the donor had recorded before his death.

"When they played me some of his music, I could finish the phrases of his songs. I could never play before, but after my transplant, I began to love music. I felt it in my heart. My heart had to play it. I told my mom I wanted to take guitar lessons, the same instrument Paul had played. His song is in me. I feel it a lot at night and it's like Paul is serenading me."

I write music myself these days, recorded on a little 8-track recorder and with the sound of a small child eagerly trying to impress their parents. I've not found my writing moving in a direction of my donor, but more introspectively about my brother, or just the mundane journey of life that can feel both equally boring and important. It's embarrassing and slightly narcissistic to admit that one of my songs is on my iTunes "most played" list. I can guarantee it wouldn't feature on anyone else's.

But it's not just about picking up an instrument and finding a new skill. For many recipients it is simply enjoying a genre of music that had no particular resonation before, such as opera and jazz.

Looking into my past I wouldn't say I have a love of classical music, but I certainly don't mind it. It formed part of my early life, like most children going through music lessons, but I probably went through a period where music become all about the rebellion of rock music. When I say "rebellion" it was actually Dire Straits. I know. My brother was the rebellious one, and how I wish it had been me.

In the early days after my transplant I did find myself going to the Royal Opera House to watch an Opera, and I used to go and see the local opera performances whenever they turned up at my local theatre, but that felt a natural extension of my musical interests. Maybe it was something more.

Even the most talented and famous amongst us can be affected by the characteristics of the donor that breathed new life into our musical souls. The R&B singer Natalie Cole, daughter of the iconic Nat King Cole, had a kidney transplant in 2009 following a battle with hepatitis C. Cole's donor was a young woman who had tragically died during child birth in El Salvador.

Despite not being able to speak Spanish, Cole decided to record an entire album in the language of her donor as a way of a tribute to the woman that had saved her life. It's not just the sentiment that Cole feels but something that runs much deeper as she told billboard.com. "I don't believe in coincidences. I believe everything happens for a reason. That this donor was from a Latin family, I feel like I'm part Latino now. That made the desire to make this record become even stronger."

It's quite a tribute and listening to the songs it is amazing to think that Natalie Cole learnt the songs phonetically. Maybe her donor is really coming out in her singing? Whatever the reason, it's a beautiful album and one to add to my collection.

So how do I work out what my donor's musical talent or taste is without discovering a hidden talent deep within my own self? It maybe needs to be something I've not played before, but something that's really chosen by my heart.

A website offers to steer users through a journey in order to find the instrument that best suits them via several questions around musical taste and skill. I try to answer everything as I think my donor would. I already had a suspicion that they may have liked R&B from my experiences after transplant when I cried at Boyz II Men, and that forms part of my response. After a few unusual questions about my "favourite animal" and if I am a "leader or a follower", I'm then presented with the kind of instrument I should be looking for. The profile suggests my donor's choice of instrument is quite different from the general population, and that I should be looking for something with a unique sound. It suggests something like a xylophone. I'm not so sure my donor wants to play the xylophone, but "unique" fits the bill and so it's off to some music shops to find a new sound.

Luckily Norwich has an abundance of independent music shops, and all nicely cluttered down one road, so I soon find myself amongst a vast variety of different instruments. Sadly this "vast variety" seems to be made up mainly of guitars and then other variations on that theme, such as the banjo or ukulele.

I was hoping to find something without strings, as I've spent too much time playing the guitar already for anything string based to feel different. The shops don't really help either as they have the feel of being as welcoming as a cat poo on a pizza. Maybe I just feel uncomfortable, and maybe my donor does too. Time to leave, and I do it with an air of dejection.

Where next then? Surely I've exhausted the immediate possibilities and I'll have to resort to my online safety net of eBay or Amazon. Damn, I was just in the mood to start and this feels a disappointment. Jennifer is with me, and as usual she wants to go and look in some antique shops for little vintage collectables so cunningly she suggests I may find something there.

The first couple of shops are a maze of bric-a-brac and vintage clothes, but it's hard to find anything musical bar the odd piano and a couple of wooden recorders that I already know how to play. We move on to a much larger shop which generally has bigger pieces of furniture and an assortment of eclectic items. I'm not feeling confident, but we move through the store with one purpose in mind.

As I make my way through a collection of old Casio style keyboards I notice a large, dusty suitcase style box over in the corner. Just appearing out of it is a set of ivory looking keys that appear as though they are attached to something much larger. I open the box and before me is an old looking, but very beautiful accordion. My eyes light and I call Jennifer over. She helps me pick it up, and with one gentle squeeze the most beautiful deep chord comes out of the box. I can feel both my head and heart wanting this, and at £55 it looks a bargain.

Jennifer is not disappointed either, finding some mustard coloured vintage cups and saucers. Today we are both winners and we are soon out of the shop clutching our new prized possessions. Some days feel a struggle but the battle makes the joy at the end of it seem so much more rich.

Once home I look at the full beauty of this old machine. Made by Laguna it has a gorgeous ice blue finish to it with a silver frame and old wooden piano keys. Some well worn but sturdy leather straps finish it off. As I place it round my chest I already feel a sense of joy just holding it in my hands. I let the left side of the accordion fall down with a gentle pull of my hand and press one of the many bass keys at my fingers. The sound is loud, deep, warm and extremely satisfying.

The next question is how much talent do I have for this instrument? It deserves someone that can make it sing like it hasn't done for a few years. I don't want to read up on how to play it, but just let my heart and soul come together and see what happens. Is it in me?

I move the bellows apart and together again, working my way around the bass buttons first. The noise is truly overwhelming but I can't seem to find any pattern to the keys at all. What I do find is that just like my harmonica you can make a fairly decent noise straight away, and the buttons clearly work on a blow and draw system.

I can hear some of the chords and try to work out where my favourite combination of C, F and G are, as I know once I get this I will start to feel more confident.

It still doesn't feel particularly intuitive, but I start to get a bit more of a structured sound, so start to try the keyboard notes on the right side of the harmonica. My keyboard playing is limited to what I manage on my iPad, so I quickly make a sound like a small child let loose on a plastic keyboard. To make matters worse I can't control what my left hand does when my right hand tries to play. This is obviously the well known male condition of not being able to multitask. I can drink a beer and watch football at the same time so I know that's applicable to me.

A few hours pass and I'm very in love with my new accordion or squeeze box, as they are affectionately known. Time for a rest and to think about getting a proper tune out of it. If I have any discernible talent, then some form of song should be the minimum standard expected.

I need something that will be simple on the keyboard, and with a few basic chords. I have made a recording of "Little Donkey" before for Jennifer, and I need something just as easy. I start to hum to myself and strangely as I try to sing "Little Donkey", I end up in a rendition of "How Much Is That Doggy in the Window". I'm not sure how that happened but it feels right.

The basic chorus I quickly pick up on the keyboard so it's just trying to put that together with the correct chords. I'm still unsure which is which chord, although through a basic combination of keyboard presses and bass button pushing I can soon get a picture. I'm just really hot, frustrated and struggling to make it all come together. I can't twiddle the knobs and push all the same buttons at once. It's proving just as difficult as my love life.

Frustration gets the better of me. It's been a long while since I had an instrument I couldn't quickly start playing, and whilst this should prove no more difficult, this skill seems beyond me at the moment. I don't so much have a "doggy in the window" but more an "annoying fly caught in the blinds". Still, no one has recorded that version so it's royalty free.

I sit down with a cup of tea and try and remember why I'm doing this. I'm just trying to see if there is a hidden talent my donor had for music. At the moment it doesn't feel as though he did, but going by how much I love the sound of the accordion and my relative surprise at owning one, I know I have something I'm going to go forward with and learn.

There might not be any natural talent here, but I've found something new to love, and without my donor I would never have gone in this direction. Maybe they were musical, or maybe they were the type of character that just liked trying new things. Maybe certain noises just appeal.

Whatever the reason, the accordion takes up a special place in my living room. It's a reminder that we should never stop learning, and it's also a reminder of my donor. Every time I look at it I shall think of him, and then after that I shall just admire how truly beautiful it is. Almost as beautiful as the act of donation itself.

Heroes, Villains and the Gift of Life

"It's the gift of life itself... You have a sense that after you've been through all of that, everything else is small. A friend of mine asked me when I told him it was a spiritual experience: "Does that mean now, that you're a Democrat?" I told him, "Well, not that spiritual.""

Dick Cheney (Former Vice President of the United States & Heart Transplant recipient)

It's a Friday and unusually for a Friday I sat down with a game in front of me. I don't own a PlayStation and I'm not one for playing one of the many additive games now found on smartphones. The game that I've removed from its rather worn box is "Guess Who?"

I would think that any parent would already know this game, and indeed most generations of family have probably played a version of it. The game has a simple objective, you just need to guess the mystery person as selected by your opponent by asking questions in turn that eliminate any of the faces that do not match the mystery person's description.

So why am I playing? And more, why on earth is a 43 year old man playing this game, on his own, on a Friday afternoon. Boredom? Maybe. Intrigue? Definitely.

I've been trying to think about all of the characteristics my donor might have had, and it has occurred to me that I don't have any feeling or conception of what my donor might look like. As a starting point, a process of elimination seemed a good idea, and "Guess Who?" offers just that.

So the first characters to fall are all the female ones, as I already know that my donor is male. Out go Maria, Betty, Sally, Sarah, Holly and Anita.

The next thing I do know is that my donor was 33 at the time of his death. He would be 52 now, so how should I visualise him? Personally I see him as a 33 year old still, but that's not a question you can ask with "Guess Who?". So next I remove all those with bald heads, as a full head of hair fits more with my vision. Out go Bill, Roger, Herman, Albert and Charles. Eleven down, thirteen to go.

What next? It was the nineties when my donor died, facial hair wasn't that popular, and for some reason an image of a bearded or moustachioed male does not spring to mind. There appears to be a lot of furry faces on "Guess Who?" That removes Mario, Hans, Frederick, Luke, Alfred and Max.

I work my way through the list, removing grey hair, glasses and people with hats, although I'm not sure why I feel so strongly against wearing something on your head. My list is further trimmed of Paul, Eric, Bernard, Victor and Joe.

So that leaves me with just two. Frank and Robert. This poses a question, and an interesting one about race. Frank is a youthful looking black man with a kindly yet quizzical face, Robert is a blue eyed white man with a long horse like face and the appearance of a banker. So do I think my heart was from someone of a different race to me? How would I even know? Even if the heart was more than a pump, people are people and our character traits are not defined by race. Even so, my feeling is towards Robert. So there we have it, in a game limited to 24 people, I see my donor as a blue eyed banker.

So why would I think like this? We are all told that it's important to find a "match" when we are on the waiting list, and we are also warned of the possibility of us rejecting the new organ. All of us look for the qualities we ourselves possess, so if you're caring you probably want a caring partner. I suspect I'm just looking for whoever is the person that most closely matches my own vision of myself. Of course I've never thought of myself as a "banker", although some comments about me have certainly sounded like that.

All transplant recipients tend to think of our donors as amazing people, the ones that saved our lives, and someone like that will always be someone of almost supernatural qualities. I spoke to a few transplant friends to see how they would describe their donor.

"My donor's my hero. She always will be"

"Two donors, don't know them but, girl 17 and man 63, selfless angels"

"I call my donor by his name, it was his choice to help save lives!"

"Zara, or Hero with a Halo"

"Husband! ;)"

"Mine is my guardian angel"

"I always say my angel xx"

It just shows how much we think of these donors, but in many respects they are just people like you and me, with families that understood the good that could come out of something so devastating. Maybe the best description of what we should call our donors comes from Sally, the mother of a donor.

"I would like Toby to be referred by his recipients to as just that by his name no more no less."

Whilst thinking through who my donor might be another story appeared in the national press that caused a huge stir. I was asked by several people about my views on it, but I wanted to stay away from the subject, it was far too sensitive for rational argument, especially if you have been affected by waiting on the transplant list.

The article first appeared in the Daily Mail on the 3rd December and concerned a heroin addict who had been given a heart transplant and subsequently had been jailed for 18 months after obtaining more than 30 convictions.

I certainly don't judge anyone's views on the story, and definitely not those of you waiting on the list or watching a loved one wait. I've been there, I do understand that the list is hard enough as it is, and that the most deserving person will always be yourself. That's how it should feel.

Working my way through the article though I couldn't help but make some observations based on my own thoughts and experiences. These are just my opinions.

The first couple of paragraphs state "Derek Gates, 38, was cleared for surgery by doctors even though his heart problems were caused by drug addiction".

The important thing to remember here is that he was "cleared by doctors". If you have ever been assessed for transplantation you will know these decisions are not made lightly, even when you seem to have everything going for you. Any drug user would have to prove themselves capable of adhering to the strict conditions doctors placed on them, and only then would they be placed on the list. So in that respect it seems fair. Doctors have to make medical judgements, they cannot make moral ones.

The statement that "even though his heart problems were caused by drug addiction" requires some analysis. Many of those people awaiting a transplant will have done things in their lives that may have contributed to their ill health. Smokers, drinkers, heavy eaters. Most of us have our vices, none of us indulged in them with the thought we would ever end up on a transplant list. So is a smoker alright, but a drinker not? Someone addicted to sugar fine, but to drugs not? Where do you draw the line? Is addiction an illness? If so is an addict really any more to blame for his health than someone picking up a virus?

Again to me the key part is that the doctors made that decision. He was unwell and he was considered suitable for transplant.

The next paragraph goes on to speak about Gates' life following transplant. "Instead of mending his ways, he responded by stepping up his criminal behaviour."

I worry about this line of thinking, as it suggests that we have been given a second chance and that we should somehow do some greater good with it. Many of the transplant patients I know do just that, and I think that's a massive tribute to the families that donate, but should it be expected that we improve our lives?

You would hope that a drug user could pull themselves out of the life they got themselves into, but it's not that simple. We should hope that all addicts can find the help they need, and with luck, find a better way to deal with their lives. That applies to every addict. We shouldn't be expecting more of someone just because they have been given a new heart. Transplantation is not easy, being a drug addict is not an easy life either. It shouldn't be surprising that you may not cope and fall back into bad habits.

I don't think I should be judged on my actions post-transplant any more than someone in good health. I don't think we should judge Gates either.

The article then increases the emotional volume by talking to recipients and family members of transplant patients. The response they give is what you would expect and I fully support their right to those opinions. One line is particularly telling, coming from a 67 year old heart transplantee. "How will the families feel of the person whose heart he inherited?"

One wonders. And I suspect it will be one of horror and disgust. The point is extremely valid, but the only reason they may know, and in fact the only reason that potentially millions of donors know is that the Daily Mail has chosen to tell them. That's extremely dangerous.

Who does this story serve? We need all the donors we can get. Many will die waiting and to the Daily Mail the goal is to highlight the sort of individual it feels shouldn't be on the list. Remove the undeserving and therefore more deserving people will live. That's the message. But all they have done is make people question why they should donate. Many might decide to remove their names from the register, many will decide that they are right not to sign up. Will someone else die because Gates is on the transplant list? Maybe. Will someone die because the story reduced donor numbers? Certainly.

Lack of donors is the real story, and the storm caused by articles like these detract from that essential message. We need more donors. With enough donors we would end up with less people who die waiting, and with luck everyone gets their chance. It would reduce the morality question and leave everyone just to get on with trying to survive as best they can.

A follow up story appeared three days later, in which the Daily Mail revealed that Gates was back awaiting a second transplant, although on reading it sounds like the Daily Mail have made this assumption based on his sister's views that the current heart was nearing the end of its lifespan.

The comments section following the article highlights just how outraged potential donors might be.

"Give a heart to someone that's gonna do something with there (sic) life or a child or someone with a family not him would be unjustified"

"Give the heart to someone more deserving"

"Such a precious gift should go to someone deserving"

"Stories like this would put people off becoming donors"

And then there are a good few comments like these ones below that I understand, but also really worry about.

"I carry a donor card and there is no way I would want my organs going to a waster like that, unfortunately we don't have a choice. Which is totally wrong, my organs, why can't I say who they go to????"

"These cases have undone all the work done by the Transplant organisations and reinforces my belief that I will never donate unless I have a say in who receives."

I started off this chapter happily wondering who my donor is, what type of person he was, how he looked and came to the conclusion I hoped he may be someone like myself.

In hoping for that I am setting an expectation about who my donor is. What if they had lived a life of crime? Maybe they had their own addictions? How would I feel then?

In many ways I am expecting exactly the same level of morality and behaviour from my donor as those potential donors want to see in their "chosen" recipients.

When I flipped down the faces of those characters that I didn't think suited my donor, I was trying to make a match that I thought was right for me, but the reality is it shouldn't matter. I needed a new heart, and if that heart was medically suitable for me then it does not matter who that came from, or their background or criminal record. Equally we can't choose to flip down the faces of those we think are not suited to an organ. If it's medically suited to them, then we have to accept that is right on medical grounds.

Somehow we need to remove the emotional aspect of the donor list, but that's very hard when you have to use emotion to encourage more donors. We happily donate our blood without worrying about who gets it, and the same should apply with our organs.

The use of emotion to encourage donation is vital, but whilst it exists we will always want to have some emotional involvement in the outcome. The most commonly used phrase to support organ donation is "the gift of life", it's highly emotive, it supports the idea of personal choice and, as with most gifts you give, it suggests something the recipient should cherish.

For me, I've used the phrase "the gift of life" thousands of times. I've used it to encourage others, to say thank you to my donor, to just explain to others what I have been through. Equally though it is probably the source of some of my guilt. Have I done enough with the gift? If someone gives you "the gift of life", can you ever do enough to say thank you? What if you grow tired of life? We've all had that present we can't throw out because we know how much it meant to the person who gave it to us. Imagine if that gift was life, and you felt it had little value for you. Depression is hard enough without feeling you owe someone to be making use of your life.

We are not going to get away from "the gift of life", but maybe we need to look more closely in society as to how we deal with organ donation. In an earlier chapter I gave my thoughts on the Welsh Assembly's move to an opt-out system. I reflected on the idea that more education is required and I hoped we could fulfil our requirements within the current opt-in system.

Sadly I think stories like the one in the Daily Mail will only serve to provide misinformation, lower donor numbers and strengthen the belief that we have a right to choose who gets our "gift".

Reflecting on it, maybe an opt-out system sets out the right message. When you are gone, if your organs are suitable, they will be used in a medical procedure to help someone else. It's not a gift, just part of a caring societies' duty. And if you are against that, if you don't want your organs used or you feel you want to have some say in where they go, then just opt-out. It's your choice, and freedom of choice is also something we should value as a society too.

So, maybe my donor was a banker, maybe he was a dealer, maybe a drug addict will get your organs. One thing is certain, if everyone left the register because they worried about it, a lot of very good, kind, family orientated people would die.

Sign up. Save a life.

Welcoming the Intruder

"An Israeli man's life was saved when he was given a Palestinian man's heart in a heart transplant operation. The guy is doing fine, but the bad news is, he can't stop throwing rocks at himself."

Jay Leno (host of NBC's The Tonight Show with Jay Leno from 1992 to 2009.)

As usual I find it impossible to find the right buttons on my remote control. I can never understand the size of these instruments of torture, when it seems to me a television requires only three basic functions, to switch it on or off, to change channel and to adjust the volume. So why does my remote need 31 buttons? And of those, which is the one to adjust the size of my picture?

Normally I'm perfectly happy with whatever picture my television presents to me, but today I have settled in to watch a film. As often is the case with me, the film is foreign and subtitled. The only downside is my television does not wish to show me the text I require in order to make this an enjoyable experience. After several frustrating button thrusts, I finally get to what I need. Now, how to go back to the beginning?

Luckily I've not missed anything, just a few opening shots set in a darkness that leaves the viewer just able to see a woman lighting a cigarette. The credits soon appear "L'intrus" or to give it's English title "The Intruder"

The opening scenes generally revolve around the main character (Sidney Trebor), a rough man in his fifties, who is seen variously roaming the French countryside naked with his two husky dogs. Very obviously a poorly man, we see him struggling with his breathing and trying to recover from a swim in the lake. My mother always warned me that if you are going to be found dead it's best to look presentable, not maybe naked with your two dogs sniffing at your corpse.

We then see Sidney cycling the countryside, feeding his dogs and having sex with an attractive, local pharmacist. So far, so French.

Then during one evening there is a disturbance, and we see our man with blood on his hands. A young man has been killed and who we assume has "intruded" on Sidney's property. Quietly, Sidney continues to go about his business despite the health problems he is clearly having. The body of the young man is eventually discovered, bloody and with a heart that is outside of his deceased body.

Now, you may be wondering, what I'm doing mentioning this seemingly perplexing movie? Certainly it's no "Ice Age 2", but stay with me, there is a reason.

What we see next is Sidney travelling to Korea and looking to organise his own black market heart transplant. He hands his medical records over to an organiser and requests that his donor be "a young man, not a woman or an old man". It's not long before we see Sidney reveal his body from the under the covers of his hotel bed, to reveal that an operation has now been performed.

Now I don't normally have an eye for detail. Small things easily pass me by, but as I watched Sidney take his medication, I was pleasantly surprised to see him use exactly the same pill organiser that I do. That was the most exciting part so far. A pill organiser.

We then learn that Sidney has other business in Korea as well. He voyages to Tahiti in a search for the son that he fathered many years previously. The rest of the film centres on his attempts to fit back in with this strange environment and the struggle of the uncertain welcome that he will receive. We also see him continue to have various difficulties with his health and the occasional concerned touch of his scar as he considers the impacts of his operation.

The end, like many arty films, is sudden, and just switches from Sidney, on what could be a boat home with his lost son, to a shot of the huskies running through the snow. I won't look for the sequel.

So why mention this? Am I just watching every film that has an element of transplantation in it? I hope not, there are quite a lot of them. The reason for watching this particular film is that it was based on a piece of work by the French philosopher Jean-Luc Nancy, and Nancy just happens to be a heart transplant patient himself.

What interested me about Nancy was how his thoughts and writing on his transplant were very different from my own, and gave me a completely different perspective on this unique operation.

Nancy describes an experience where an intruder (l'intrus) forcibly enters the body without its right to enter or being admitted in the first place. An intruder whose presence is unexpected and is always going to remain "foreign". All my thoughts previously had been on how welcome the "gift" had been. Nancy, though, was speaking about the concept of the body and the intrusion of illness, and his words actually felt like the opening of an envelope containing a guilty secret.

L'intrus was originally published in 2000, containing Nancy's thoughts on his heart transplant that he received ten years previously. The film adaption, which is based on his writing, came out in 2004. Much of the film's elements are about the killing of "the intruder" and the feelings of trying to gain acceptance and find the familiar in a foreign land are clearly metaphors for his own body's battle with this new organ.

Nancy describes how his own heart had begun to fail him. His heart was simply giving up and rejecting him and to that extent was becoming a stranger, an intruder itself in the body it no longer seemed to want to be a part of.

The process of being placed on the transplant list is met with one of both surprise at the assessment of suitability, and also the moral questions that being on the list raises. Who decides? It's a confusing place to find yourself. Nancy states *"From the first, my survival is inscribed in a complex process woven through with strangers and strangeness."*

Thoughts also centre on something that I have always pondered myself. Why do we strive so much to ensure 'survival'. What does it mean to survive, and is quantity more important than quality? I've always felt that my destiny was to die aged 23 or 24, but technology and intelligent people stepped in and changed what was natures will. Nature certainly didn't want me walking around with the heart of another human, and at great expense. So why do we do it?

As a transplantee, surviving also means a medical regime that lowers our immune system in order to accept the new organ, and in this respect Nancy likens the process to that of becoming a foreigner to oneself. Not only is the new organ a "foreign" object, but the medication means the recipient becomes a stranger to their own bodies immune system's identity. Other foreigners then appear in the form of shingles and other virus's that have laid dormant through the years.

It all feels very lonely and confusing to me. The body forced to accept this organ, the losing of identity and of being a stranger even to yourself. Most transplant patients probably wouldn't speak like this, but I'm pretty sure the majority would identify with Nancy's feelings.

"I feel it distinctly; it is much stronger than a sensation: never has the strangeness of my own identity, which I've nonetheless always found so striking, touched me with such acuity. "I" has clearly become the formal index of an unverifiable and impalpable system of linkages. Between myself and me there has always been a gap of space-time: but now there is the opening of an incision and an immune system that is at odds with itself, forever at cross purposes, irreconcilable."

So are the realities of transplantation that we will forever have a stranger contained within us? An unwelcome presence with all its own trauma and history, equally lost in this new strange host environment? One woman clearly doesn't think so. And that woman is Julie Motz.

"Now I want you to talk to your new heart and welcome it into your body. Tell it that you are just as excited about its information and its history as you hope it will be about yours. Tell it that you intend to honour and to use everything it knows. And know, Paul, that you are giving

146

this new heart a life that it would never have had without you."

To the average person the above quote may not impart any real feeling or emotion, indeed if anything it might just seem a little odd and jarring with our natural understanding of the order of things. The words suggest that life goes much further than our comprehension, and whilst I don't subscribe to that view, I was astounded it was a viewpoint I had never thought about before.

Through much of the writing of this book I've looked at things from a perspective of guilt. Guilt that my donor died, and that his death ultimately lead to my survival. Those words, though, have given me something new to think about; that this heart was going to cease beating and all life was going to end. I was just the lucky person in need of a heart, and I could offer it a new home, a new place to beat. Why have I never heard or thought this before? Who was the person behind this alternative perspective?

I'd stumbled across Julie Motz, an energy healer, on one of my many searches on the internet as I delved deeper, trying to find more stories relating to cellular memory. Much of the information available are comments on either Pearsall's research or Sylvia's story, and at first glance this blog appeared to be no different, until some new names appeared. Those of Julie Motz and Dr Mehmet Oz.

I'll be the first to admit that energy-healing is not something I have ever experienced, and I've probably closed myself off to the idea of alternative healing, based on the long history of trust I have had to place on traditional medicine.

Here though, was a story of a non-traditional healer being allowed to work in the operating theatre, and during such major operations as heart transplants. I can't imagine this happening within the NHS, but maybe it does? Certainly it seemed unusual, so surely a transplant unit had decided there was some benefit, but what sort of surgeon would be open to the ideas of energy healing?

Being from the UK, the name Mehmet Oz meant very little to me, just another doctors name linked to the world of transplantation that I've become so fascinated by. To Americans though, he is the most high profile Doctor on the planet, with his own "The Dr Oz Show", currently one of the highest rated daily television shows in the nation, and who was described by Oprah Winfrey in 2004 as "America's doctor". Oz currently has a following of 3.2 million on his twitter feed alone. That's quite a profile. More than just another TV personality, many heart transplant patients owe their lives to Dr Oz.

The profile of Julie Motz was much lower, but it was her story that intrigued me the most. She was not the kind of person you might suspect would become a healer, coming from a very intellectual and scientific family. Her brother became a doctor and indeed Julie started out in a career as a documentary filmmaker.

During an acrobatics class, Julie injured her back and with western medicines being unable to provide an answer she turned to acupuncture and other therapies with limited or little success. It was at a friend's dinner party where the strength of energy healing first revealed its true powers.

The host of the party had healed herself of ovarian cancer, with a macrobiotic diet and a form of energy healing called Rieki. Impressed, Julie mentioned her back and the hostess began some work by putting her hands on Julie's shoulder. As she worked, Julie got an image of her mother with her hand raised to slap her across the face when she was three. The host then raised Julie's hand to remove the pain, and with it Julie burst into tears, the image faded and the pain was completely removed.

Clearly fascinated by this discovery, Julie began taking a real interest in how emotions and traumatic memories could be stored in the body, and how that would translate into very real, physical pain. She then signed up for a degree in Public Health at Columbia, connecting with doctors at the hospital, including Dr. Oz.

Her initial involvement with Dr Oz involved hypnosis experiments with sixty coronary bypass patients, including a control group, and a remaining group that were taught self-hypnosis. The aim of the trial was to reduce the pain and discomfort many patients went through post-operatively. Results were favourable and Julie was allowed to focus on some of Dr Oz's other patients, specifically those with transplants.

Soon Motz was a presence in the operating theatre too. She had worked extensively with a patient called George, who was on the transplant waiting list and being kept alive by a mechanical pump. The building up of trust meant that Motz, being there during surgery, would be valued by both patient and surgeon alike.

During surgery, when Dr Oz finally removes George's old heart, a feeling of sadness overwhelms Motz and she feels unable to know if the sorrow is George's, the new hearts, or both of them. The same feeling comes across as the new heart is handed over to Dr Oz, but being unable to hold the precious organ, Motz is still uncertain of what the cause might be.

Realising that George's life has revolved around taking care of other people, she senses he is trying to protect his new heart from his sadness, a welcome maybe, but not an open one. During a post-operative visit, George is asked to tell his new heart everything about his life, including how he has been hurt. One week later, and George is a happy patient, his blood pressure stabilising not long after his conversation with Motz. That night George had told his life story to his new heart, and the effects had been positive.

As I read through Motz's own book, describing her relationship with more patients like George, I find myself increasingly liking and believing in this woman. The photo on the front cover of "Hands of Life" is of an attractive, slender and kindly lady, dressed in blue scrubs and looking like the kind of professional you'd seek out when you want reassurance.

I don't often cry when reading books, in fact I would say I probably never do, but as I read through another of the stories detailing the tense atmosphere during transplant surgery, I found myself uncontrollably moved. The tears were not out of fear for what might happen, but out of the sheer kindness and care Motz had for her patients and what they were going through.

The patient was called Susan, a former day care worker who was held with great affection by the children she had worked with. During Motz's time with Susan, before the transplantation, it became clear that there is a lot of sadness in Susan's life stemming from her own treatment as a child.

When the transplant finally comes and Susan is opened up by Dr Oz, Motz can sense feelings of an angry little girl, yet there is some sense of relief when Dr Oz asks how the patient is doing.

The heart is finally brought in, the donor having been involved in a car crash. The mother of the donor sadly at the wheel during the accident that left her daughter dead.

"Remembering the image that had come to me at the ice chest, I realised that the heart was afraid to get angry or show aggression in any way. It was afraid that anger would lead to death, as it did in the car, mirroring Susan's own fear that anger brings only punishment"

Feeling that both Susan and the new heart need to get angry, Motz does something that she hadn't done up until now for fear of embarrassment.

"I held my hand up in the air, above the sheet marking off the sterile field, and sent energy directly into Susan's new heart. 'Give up despair, and let hope come into your chest,' I told her. 'Fight for what you want.' I felt the heart perk up. Dr Oz announced that it was beating regularly and she was out of danger."

I'm not entirely sure what went on in those moments, but I am convinced that the work Motz was doing played a part. As a patient I know that I can still register voices and conversation when I'm not fully conscious. When I have my operations and I'm having a local anaesthetic, I'm always grateful for the conversation with my doctor, part reassurance and part idle chit chat. An operation like a transplant is going to be hugely stressful, and Motz's soothing voice and care must shine through like a huge beacon.

Motz doesn't believe that consciousness is just localised to the brain, with personality and memory existing within all the cells that make us all up. This belief would certainly allow for the storage of memories to appear within donor organs and then be passed to the recipient. Motz states that "memory precedes the formation of the nervous system and must therefore exist on a cellular level".

Certainly Motz gets to experience what this effect has on some of the patients she works for, and like many people's experiences following transplant you can either choose to believe them or just put it down to the psychological and pharmaceutical changes that a patient goes through.

"Kenneth's new heart seemed unusually happy, and when I saw him a few days after surgery, an incredible brightness shone in his eyes, almost as if some other, much younger and more animated person were peering out from inside him. I later discovered that he had gotten the heart of a twenty-five year old girl, who, he speculated, had been into a much healthier lifestyle than his own. A former greasy-food addict, he now found himself mysteriously craving salads."

If Jean-Luc Nancy was experiencing an intruder, Julie Motz would certainly be there trying to make the experience a far more welcoming one. There is a lot we do not understand, and both Nancy and Motz offer very interesting viewpoints.

One thing is certain, if I ever go through another transplant, I'd like Julie Motz to be in the operating theatre with me. At your most vulnerable, you need someone that cares. Julie Motz cares.

The following is a poem written by Julie Motz.

Between Lives

You come with your great, broken hearts,
scarred with the blood of a thousand weeping wounds.
It is not your courage which needs mending,
nor your love -
only some small, hidden, sorrowful part
which has run rampant in your being,
shredding the fibres of life in its unspoken agony.

They search for it everywhere,
in all the vital fluids

and in the ailing flesh
which you offer so generously,
so hopefully,
to the testing and probing
of physicians' hurried minds.

You know that finally you must be touched
on the inside,
where you yourselves have not been allowed to reach.
You hope that each finger of the surgeon's hands
contains a thousand brains
and the love of a thousand hearts.
You dare to believe that it does.

Do you know that he comes into your bodies seeking love,
and knowledge he can find no other place?
Do you know the reverence and the mystery of his
entering?

You open yourselves to show him the treasures of your
being,
each chamber chanting the music of your life.
He senses the harmonies they are straining for
even as his eyes record the chaos of his own intrusion
and the more subtle disorder which has summoned him to
this place.

You live again, even as you sleep, all the old, losing battles

where your child's faith rode forth, unarmed.
All the unheard crying is here,
and the things which wore your hearts to pieces
as your brain observes the memory
in silent rage.

Then it comes for each of you -
the moment to lift your dreams from loneliness,
to rescue hope
and put it in the mouth of your new heart.

Test 4 - Boyz II Men

"And then I hear this song -- it was Sade. And I'm just crying. Six months later, Brady's mom called and introduced herself and told me I had her son's heart. We got to talking and she said,'Well, his favourite singer was Sade.'"

Bill Wohl (heart transplant patient whose donor was a 36-year-old, Sade listening, Hollywood stuntman)

Internet shopping has many advantages, although I'm fairly certain my postman will disagree with that statement after my recent Christmas activity. The main advantage in this instance though, is the privacy it provides, well if you exclude the fact that my shopping preferences will be logged on Amazons huge database. Today I am browsing "Boyz II Men". Frightening.

Why am I spending my time staring into Amazons darker corners? Well I need to test those two strange incidents from my time in intensive care and recovery, just after my own operation back in 1994.

My unusual choice of sustenance, post operation, of rhubarb yogurt may say more about my donor than me. Take heart transplant patient David Waters from Australia, who found he had a sudden craving for Burger Rings, a corn based snack, immediately after his operation. Two years afterwards, after an e-mail exchange with his donor's family, David was to discover that the very same snack was eaten daily by his donor, Kaden. Could it be that rhubarb yogurt had also been my donors favourite milk based product?

The second incident was the odd reaction I felt as my tears flooded out as I listened to Boyz II Men play "End of the Road" over the radio. Would my donor's musical preferences really have that kind of impact? The mother of a 17 year old donor spoke in Pearsall's report about her son's love of the violin and his tragic death from a drive-by shooting.

"Our son was walking to violin class when he was hit.

Nobody knows where the bullet came from, but it just hit him and he fell. He died right there on the street hugging his violin case. He loved music and his teachers said he had a real thing for it. He would listen to music and play along with it. I think he would have been at Carnegie Hall someday, but the other kids always made fun of the music he liked."

According to the recipient's wife, her husband was far from interested in classical music before and actually hated any music of that genre. Now though it seems as though it's become a comfortable and happy part of his life.

"One more thing I should say: he's driving me nuts with the classical music. He doesn't know the name of one song and never, never listened to it before. Now, he sits for hours and listens to it. He even whistles classical music songs that he could never know. How does he know them?"

Strange indeed.

As I return to my search I am faced with a choice of eleven DVD options, one of which seems to come in at the rather high price of £78.17. Who is this for? Are there Boyz II Men addicts out there and dealers willing to exhort them from their hard earned money?

The first one I view is called "Motown Live - A Journey Through Hitsville USA", with the boys performing a range of Classic Motown numbers. On the list at number 11 is the one song I'm interested in, "End of the Road". Hmm, I'll have to go through ten songs to get to that, but a review by "Stas" states "I can see it every day, but I will never tire of doing it!". High praise, and I wonder if "Stas" is anything like my donor.

Next we have "Live in South Korea". From the title I am assuming that the boys are performing their songs live again, and not that this is a documentary as they choose to see out their days living under the South Korean flag. I suppose you could hope that's the case, but sadly it is another run down of much the same songs. The one bonus is that during "It's So Hard to Say Goodbye to Yesterday" they sing into microphones that are broadcast into North Korea. If anything could bring down communist rule it's got to be Boyz II Men.

The final offering I look at is called "Millenium" oddly released in 2004. Maybe they should have gone for

"Millenium Plus Four", which would reflect both the year and the number of the boys. I'm getting a bit more of a feel for them now. This is just a collection of videos and doesn't mention "End of the Road" and it only gets four stars.

I plump for the Motown DVD, it's well reviewed, especially by "Stas", and it's also the cheapest. It's interesting to note what else customers have bought. If you have ever purchased on Amazon you'll know that they generally get it right in serving you up what you may like, so maybe this is some further insight into what my donor may have liked.

There is Stevie Wonder, Alexander O'Neil, good old Whitney Houston and some lady called Brandy. I've never heard of Brandy, but her album was released in 1994. Maybe it's worth a shot too? Looking at the tracks they could be made for transplantation, with tracks such as "Brokenhearted", "I'm Yours", "Always On My Mind" and "Give Me You". It's in my basket.

The next search is a little harder as I need to find some samples of rhubarb yogurt, and since that morning in intensive care, I don't think I've ever bought any. Does anyone make this? Luckily it seems everyone does. Rachel's has an organic version, there is a Muller Light one (sadly no corner), Shape has a "rhubarb crumble" flavoured one. Do I want "flavoured" and if I do, do I want it crumble flavoured. What's wrong with just crumble? Get with the times Shape people. Then there is Waitrose with its "refreshing and creamy champagne rhubarb yogurt"; now that sounds like a winner.

I make a plan to head down to the local Waitrose and let them fleece me of my money in exchange for something that is technically gone off milk, but is still both "refreshing" and "creamy".

Its a few days until I finally make the trip, but it's not without its disappointments. First of all I find the yoghurt, but along with the words "refreshing" and "creamy" it also has the words "produced in a factory handling nuts". This is bad news. Along with my other ailments I am also highly allergic to nuts. I carry an Epipen and I generally hope not to use it. My rhubarb yoghurt of choice needs rethinking. Most of the other yoghurts I look at have the same basic problem, and in the end I am forced to settle for Rachel's Organic. Thank you Rachel, I do trust you are both organic and nut free.

I get to the checkout with four items in my basket. I'd also been swayed by some onion bhaji's, some tuna for lunch and I needed some sweetcorn. The nice Waitrose lady scans them through with a smile and then asks me for £10.49. I look to see what else I might have accidentally bought. Maybe some wine, or some expensive cut of meat. No, nothing. Just my four items. I hand over £20 and the lady kindly counts back my change for me in a style that reminded me of being at school. I've been robbed in a very middle class way.

Back home my DVD has arrived in a sealed white envelope that hid my guilty secret from the prying eyes of my postman. I did actually take it from him dressed only in a towel, so luckily he was as keen to get away as I was to make a swift exchange.

I open up the DVD to check that everything is in place, and to discover what treats lay in store for your average Boyz II Men fan. I'm immediately drawn to the accompanying leaflet. The front cover has a picture of the venue for the gig, showing the electronic billboard advertising the "Boyz". What intrigues me is the date. It's shown as July 17, one day before my transplant anniversary. I can hear you all saying "well it's not even the date! It's the day before", and yes, you are right, but it still adds to the sense of the occasion. Well it does to me.

I take the disc from its packaging and slide it into my DVD player. Goodness, we are straight in! No warnings about re-sale or distribution. Clearly there is no need. Just the main menu with a picture of the boys resplendent in pin-striped suits all pointing at each other and looking as though they are in sweet harmony. I get the options of playing each song individually or all the way through. I select "play all".

I have a little history and interview with Boyz II Men. They certainly are all about the music. And they are building up to what I am about to witness. I hope it's worth it.

As I wait I pick up my rhubarb yogurt. I haven't had this pass my lips since I was in intensive care. Well, I've had yogurt, but not the rhubarb kind. I'm trying to go back a little to that time, and I must admit it's hard whilst three pin-striped men are shouting "say yeah". I did of course. "Yeah". There are definite pieces of real organic rhubarb, but as the first spoonful reaches my taste buds, I'm slightly underwhelmed. More yogurt, maybe a little bland. The big "pow" I was expecting didn't materialise. Maybe it just needs more than one spoonful.

I have been warned however that the journey I'm about to take will have me "out of my seat" and moving "whatever I want to". It does remind me I was meant to put my washing in the washing machine. Maybe not what they had in mind, and I refocus.

Ok. I will admit it. My foot is literally tapping to "The Tracks of My Tears". I'm settling in. Rhubarb is going down, this must be what it's like to be hormonal. I quite like it.

We've moved onto "War", it's all very upbeat now. Before it started we were invited to "put your hands in the air like this". I always wonder why we need the "like this"? How many ways are there to put your hands in the air? Bank robbers don't use the "like this" part, they assume you'll know what they mean. Maybe next time you are held up, when you're asked to put your hands in the air, ask "How?", when they say "like this", just run.

I am enjoying this, more than I care for. I'm singing along with "Easy", I'm smiling, I feel at home and very at ease with myself. The song was slightly spoiled in that it started with one of the boys on the keyboards, but for the second verse he stood up front, clearly giving away the fact the keyboard part is being played by someone else. Their voices are smoothly enjoyable. Keep to what you are good at fellas.

I've finished my yogurt. I'm still not really getting any sense of emotion or real desire for it. This is what I wanted most of all when I came round from my operation. Maybe my brain was a little confused and just threw out the first two words it could think of. There is nothing wrong with Rachel's Organic Rhubarb Yogurt. I'd buy it again, but I just thought I might feel more. I stick a bit more in my bowl just in case.

We are getting close to the big moment for me, and I'm hoping it's not a rhubarb moment. I'm hoping I'll get something from "End of the Road". The boys are clearly building up to it as they are busy handing out red roses to just about any adoring hand proffered to them from the audience. Oh hold on, we have a special guest. It is the one and only Brian McNight. Yes. I thought that too. If this is a journey through Motown, they've taken a wrong turning.

Ok, this is it. I sit back, relax and pump my volume up to 45 (for a Sony, that's apparently quite loud).

Wow.

Well that was odd.

From the first few words I felt a shiver through my body, the hairs all down my arms seemed to have a static charge and there was a real sense that emotion was coming from somewhere quite deep. I almost tried to pull things back a little, but as they burst into the chorus, my eyes just welled up with water. No gushing, nothing uncontrollable, just a desire to let something out. And I'm listening to Boyz II Men for goodness sake. This isn't even my music. But it's there, it's that same feeling, I'm being dragged back and the "End of the Road" is taking me there.

I can feel my heart beating harder. Like it wants to escape. I take a few deep breaths. The crowd roars its approval, and I can sense why.

We are finishing off with a Boyz II Men classic of "Motownphilly", which I remember too, but I'm still trying to calm down as the crowd works itself into a frenzy. Where is that damn yogurt? Sod it, the rhubarb wasn't working anyway. The closing credits start to roll whilst we are still in full swing. An hour has passed and it's been both enjoyable and more emotional than I imagined. Thank you Boyz II Men.

So there we have it. I have no doubt in my mind that there is no real hidden desire for rhubarb yogurt, and I don't think the reason I wanted it after my operation was due to some "cellular" preference from my donor. It doesn't do anything for me, and I'm not going to be eating it again in a hurry.

There is, though, something in this whole "End of the Road" thing. It's out of my control and all the feelings it brings out in me comes from a completely different place. Is this my donor? Is this his music? I really don't know, but clearly it takes me back to the time of my operation, and a whole host of emotions are stored there. I still don't know why I would cry to it in the first place, but if cellular memory truly exists then you would have to put your money on this being a "memory". One day I hope to get the answer.

As I ponder my thoughts there is one last thing to do before calling an end to the afternoon. Brandy. No, it's not that I need a stiff drink after all that pent up emotion, it's Brandy the singer, and her album from 1994.

I slip it into the DVD player and settle back to some light R&B grooves. Actually that might not be an accurate description, but you might be able to tell I'm no music critic. I start to tidy things away. I have two-thirds of a 500g yogurt left. I suspect I would throw it out, but I'm reminded of the value I needed to get from my £10.49 basket of goods. It goes in the fridge. Near the back.

Brandy is fairly relaxing and I can see why Boyz II Men fans might be buying this as well, it like the come down after the excitement of the gig. It's probably what I need.

I think back to the review on Amazon by "Stas". Could I watch "Motown Live - A Journey Through Hitsville USA" every day and not get bored? Probably not, but maybe every other day, and maybe somewhere me and "Stas" could sit and sing along as the Boyz hand out their roses to the crowd. Maybe we would even "put our hands in the air like this."

I hope so. I think my donor would.

Depression

"More than 100 people are involved in a transplant operation... and we can't waste time and resources if there is a chance the caretakers aren't up for an awesome responsibility."

Leonard Lee Bailey (performed the first xenotransplantation procedure in 1984, when he placed the heart of a baboon into the chest of "Baby Fae")

"He appears to be a generally anxious personality and quite introspective and there seem to be a number of psychological issues relating to survivor guilt, fears of intimacy etc."

And so the letter continued to summarise my life, my internal struggles, my fears and failures laid on three pages in black and white. It only reflected the hour's conversation I had with the psychiatrist at my transplant unit, but reading it back I felt nothing other than shame.

It's hard to admit that you are not coping, especially when you have already come so far, further than you imagined would be possible. Shouldn't you just be enjoying life, celebrating, living. Second chance and all. Well I am, just sometimes, like everyone, I need a little help.

So what are the issues that have brought me to this point? Well I am anxious, that's very true, and everything that's laid out in this letter is maybe something that many transplant patients go through?

So what was said in that letter? Should I really feel as bad as I do first reading through it? Well this is what it has to say.

"Described anxiety in the context of coming up to the 20th anniversary of his transplant. He described "an awareness of statistics of life expectancy""

Times change. Or at least I hope they do. When I had my assessment for transplant, I was having my final discussion with the chap in charge of the programme. I was 23 years of age, having just lost my brother to this illness I now discovered I had too. I was already on the ropes. We discussed life expectancy and how a transplant was not a cure, and as we chatted about what to expect post-transplant I was told "we lose 10% of our patients each year, it's like playing Russian Roulette, each year you'll put a gun to your head, pull the trigger and hope it's not you."

Now, I don't know about you, but that had a profound effect on me, and I'm sure it's not the language that is used today, but it's stayed with me. And the newsletter that used to be sent out 6 monthly to patients had a "goodbye" section, with the names of those sadly not making it any further. Russian roulette, with the names of those that took a bullet.

"He said that his anxiety about life expectancy has impacted on a number of areas in his life, relationships in particular."

I suppose I can put a positive spin on that and say that I seem to do alright in finding some nice partners, but of course they could form a little club by now, and I suspect they would all have the same things to say about me. I worry too much. I swing between talking long-term and then acting short-term. Despite it being their choice to be in the relationship, I start pushing them away as things get closer, in my head because I'm fearful of what happens to them when I'm gone.

It's illogical and irrational. I know.

"He said he has always been an anxious person."

The way this sounds, it's as though I sit there all day worrying about life. I doubt many of my friends would see me that way, I'm generally seen as a relaxed, easy going character. Maybe too much for my bosses at work. Anxiety is a background noise, it's the quiet hum on the radio playing in the kitchen of my life.

As a child I suffered quite severe asthma attacks, hospitalised a few times, and often sat with my mother at night, a boiling kettle providing steam as I tried to regain my breathing. My body seemed to control me. I felt I had to battle it.

Then came epilepsy as a teenager. I had a couple of fits, once on Christmas Eve at home and one at school in front of all my classmates. I'd felt the world swimming before it happened, I was there but in a dream-like state, then I awoke in the sick room, exhausted. Once again, my body seemed to control me. It was in charge.

One of my favourite films is "Control" about the life of Ian Curtis of the punk band Joy Division. Ian embarks on fame just as he is diagnosed with epilepsy. Along with coping with fame and an extra-marital affair, Ian seems to struggle with how his epilepsy controls him and strikes at any given moment. No-one can know what went through his mind when he decided to hang himself, but I relate to the sense of control that action must have given him. Finally he was in charge.

On that point the letter also reads "there was no evidence of suicidal ideation or psychotic symptoms." I have had suicidal thoughts in the past, most notably after a friend committed suicide himself, but I couldn't do that to my friends, family or my donor.

"He feels that he didn't deal with his brother's death at the time because his own health became a major issue."

Adrian. Six letters, quite short and easy to say. Easy, except I never really said it. People I spoke to about my brother had to ask if he had a name. I never used it, it was like my brain just didn't want to accept he existed. My brother was a made up character in my mind, one I could deal with. Adrian was locked away elsewhere.

Waiting for my own transplant, with all that uncertain future I didn't want to accept what can happen, or maybe what was meant to happen to me if it wasn't for getting more time. Adrian became ill quickly. His death gave me more time, and to me the two felt linked. One of us was always going to go first.

"His father died of a brain tumour. His parents split up when in his early twenties after the death of his brother. He had one sibling, his brother who died of dilated cardiomyopathy."

We all have our family problems, and I honestly don't think mine are any worse or better than other people's. It's just part of life, at some point your parents are going to die; many people suffer huge loss on the journey through life. If they didn't we wouldn't have donors.

What I will say though, is that a lot came in a few very short years, and I certainly think that impacted on everything else I did going forward. As I've mentioned, I have no trust in my body. Adrian's and my father's death were very real reminders that we have no control over our destinies.

"He himself appears to have developed panic attacks shortly after his brother's death and this went on for six to seven months. He described feelings of guilt at his survival at that time and significant health anxiety."

Guilt. That's the word I would pick out. Guilt has been there on many levels. On the very first level it's the fact I had a lot of joy in myself when Adrian became ill. He'd never let my asthma stop me in anything; teasing, pushing, but in a brotherly way. When he was first sick it was a chance to get my own back. Get over it, weakling. He vomited blood and I went into his room and said kindly, "you'll be dead in two weeks." To be fair, it took three.

I should be clear here though, Adrian spoke to me in his final days in hospital, "You know you said I'd have two weeks to live, you were right." He looked at me and I held his hand. He knew I needed to hear it, and I'm grateful for his kindness when I can't even imagine what he must have felt like.

On another level, why, when my body already had so many weaknesses, didn't my heart give up first? Why when Adrian was so strong, did he suffer a fate that meant he had no time to find a donor? And if one of us was going to have a transplant, wasn't Adrian much better suited to what you have to go through. I doubt Adrian would be writing this book, he'd be winning gold at the World Transplant Games.

On the final level, guilt for my donor, something that is painfully clear through the chapters already written.

"He said that he is a bit more distracted and irritable but did not feel subjectively depressed."

Am I depressed? I don't know. I've never considered myself to be depressive; more thoughtful yet ultimately positive. Maybe that's just the image I try to project, as clearly I have one or two problems coping. But does that make me depressed?

Core symptoms of depression are listed on various websites as:

Persistent sadness or low mood. This may be with or without weepiness.

Marked loss of interest or pleasure in activities, even for activities that you normally enjoy.

I certainly can relate to having a persistent sadness, so much so that I've begun to embrace it. It feels a close friend and a state I'm actually more comfortable in. My interests remain strong, but the amount of pleasure I get from them has been slowly ebbing. More time has been spent focusing on my troubles.

Other symptoms are listed briefly as:

Disturbed sleep.

Change in appetite.

Fatigue (tiredness) or loss of energy.

Agitation or slowing of movements.

Poor concentration or indecisiveness.

Feelings of worthlessness, or excessive or inappropriate guilt.

Recurrent thoughts of death.

Certainly the last two on the list are something I'm much aware of, and the rest are common to me, but mainly I suspect through the medication I take, so may not count in any diagnosis.

It probably needs a professional to know, and obviously I'm already on that path, so in my mind, I'm doing the right thing in seeking help.

So should I feel that shame? Well yes, even after a few reads and writing this out, I still have that overriding sense that I'm letting down the transplant community. I've let the side down. There is much in the letter I haven't shared here, and mainly as I think people still will judge me. And that is shameful.

One little statement in the letter though, didn't fill me with shame, guilt or sadness. It was included near the end of the letter and I wasn't really sure why it was there. On what is essentially a medical letter, do you add any descriptive colour?

"He presents as a casually dressed man who was pleasant and cooperative with a reactive affect."

Casually dressed. Now, I made a little effort that day, but of course I was unaware of the professional etiquette of meeting a psychiatrist. I could have worn my work suit, but surely that would have made me look like some kind of psychopath, equally coming dressed in my pyjamas might have hinted at depression a little easily. So I popped on my cream cotton trousers and a suitable checked shirt. I didn't shave, but was bearded. Luckily the beard does not get a mention in the letter, my mother would have her own shame at that one.

At least I'm now aware that my appearance is going to be an important factor in these meetings and I've made plans to hire out a Pink Panther outfit for the next one. Let's see what they write on a letter then hey.

"This informally dressed man in Pink Panther costume was quite euphoric and responded in nods to all my questions."

Transplantation, organ donation, loss of family members and being on the waiting list are at times going to be difficult for anyone. Just the normality of life can be hard to handle, and sometimes as people we struggle just to get through it. Some words on the health website on depression are important to remember.

"You may 'bottle up' your symptoms from friends and relatives. However, if you are open about your feelings with close family and friends, it may help them to understand and help."

I think I've done that. Certainly I should be telling those closest to me, rather than writing it in the pages of this book, but at least they'll know. And hopefully there is someone else reading this who feels some of the things I do. I hope it helps in some small way.

The letter is roll call of the problems that have brought me to this place, but in doing that it only shows one dimension of my character, and the side I need help with. What it doesn't show is my achievements, but as I start to wind down on my sofa it's a good time to remind myself of my outstanding attributes.

One of six professional ball boys looking after Norwich City during seasons 83-85, proficient in both single and multi-ball situations.

Was a leading footwear model, described by some as having "probably the best feet it's possible to measure for a show fitting." His feet are currently retired, but open to opportunities.

Has recorded two albums and one single entitled "Waiting to Get Better", "The Homecoming EP" and the single "Christmas Crackers". Reviewed favourably, with a quote from my mother "Is that you?"

Medallist in the transplant games of 1995, 1996, 1997 and 1998. Interviewed by Radio Norfolk at trackside following a stand out 7th place finish in the 100m heats, stated "I've pulled a muscle in training so may have to give the 400m a miss."

Has a plaque in his name at Bristol Zoo's "Walk of Fame" in association with Mama Bear's Day Nursery and Pre-School. Ok, actually it's for Mark Watson the comedian, but I had the name first and I can still claim ownership. Try and stop me if you can Mark Watson.

So there you have it. A casually dressed 43 year old man, who may or may not be depressed, lies back on his sofa, takes a sip from a glass of port and taps his foot to the sounds of "The Dexateens".

I still find the letter hard to look at, and I'm still not happy, but I've taken those first steps to improving things.

No shame in that.

A Question of Sex

"Love is the answer, but while you are waiting for the answer, sex raises some pretty good questions."

Woody Allen (actor, director, comedown and playwright)

Type the words "sex" and "transplant" into Google and you'll be met with the opportunity for some gender reassignment surgery. Nothing wrong in that, but when you've already had a major organ replaced by another one, it seems a bit excessive to take it that one step further. Better to add the word "heart" to the search engine, and suddenly more relevant information is available. Phew.

So how much do you discuss your sex life? Even if it is a lot, then you are probably only framing it in a positive light, which could be very different to the dim light you may choose to perform in. What we don't seem to discuss is the problems, and as a transplant patient there is bound to be the odd issue. Well I hope so, otherwise I'm the only one. Am I? Ah.

One of the stranger statistics I found on my search was this one from the Johns Hopkins University School of Medicine in Baltimore, Maryland. In researching relationships in heart transplant patients, they found that there was a 15% improvement in the 5-year survival rate amongst patients who were married. Maybe if you are on the transplant list, you should consider getting hitched first. They also showed improved statistics for those living closer to the transplant centre. Think I'd rather move, than get married.

The British Heart Foundation also provides useful tips on sex after a transplant. Good old fashioned British advice just as we like it.

"Use the same common-sense approach to having sex again as you do to building up your other general physical activities."

So, some form of training is advisable. Probably best to ensure you have the right equipment, make sure you stretch first and to keep up motivation maybe think about joining a club. I'll have a look and see if there is anything local.

"Sex is just as safe as other equally energetic forms of physical activity or exercise."

Maybe they haven't seen some of the injuries apparently caused during a simple sex session. Variously listed as broken penises, muscle strains, rug burns, slipping over (those of you in the shower at the time), lodged objects (yes!) and of course heart attacks. Safe. I don't think so.

"Find a position which is comfortable for you, remembering not to put your chest wound under too much pressure."

Important that it is comfortable for you. Don't worry about your partner who is probably aching and bent over getting a rug burn. Oh and of course, please don't get anything "lodged".

"Try not to be too energetic at the start of your sexual activity."

Pace yourself. Remember it's a marathon not a sprint. If you have gotten yourself sponsored with payment by the mile then you have taken the concept too far. Personally I like to put the energy in at the beginning, or the end as most partners find it.

"If you are not sure when you can start having sex, talk to your transplant team or your GP."

Now I am presuming they mean before you've considered having sex. If you find yourself lying on the bed with your partner on top of you, I would suggest you are ready, but please do call your GP. They may even want to stay on the line to ensure your continued safety.

In reality, the British Heart Foundation is just saying if you feel up for it then go for it. Just don't go jumping from the wardrobe too early on. What's missing though seems to be advice on the real concerns many patients may have.

Looking back again over that list of side effects from all the medication, the years of ill health, the blood pressure problems, it's going to affect performance, and we all need reassurance.

During my search I came across a presentation that had been put together by the Pennsylvania State College of Medicine entitled "Sex After Transplant". It's an interesting document, both in its content and its style. I'm not sure who it was aimed at, but it reminded me a little of my school days (no giggling at the back).

What we learn, and the important thing here is that sexual problems are common after transplant, with issues that affect libido, erectile dysfunction and fertility. All good so far.

Next a survey is highlighted to show that out of 71 male transplant patients, many were experiencing issues mainly with erectile dysfunction that had been present during ill health but had worsened since transplant. Now, oddly, many of these patients reported that their partner's libido had *increased* post-transplant. Maybe they were expecting a partner with a new lease of life? Maybe they had been holding back when their partner was ill? But how frustrating is that? You come back to a partner that now wants to play "hunt the sausage" every day, and you've got a penis that is working less well than before. Still, this is helpful to share.

Then it turns a little odder. The next slide is some advice on "how to put the romance back into your sex life after transplant". It is important to remember they have used the word "romance". Yet they have coupled this with an image of a magnifying glass. Confused? Me too. Unless we are going to be using it to hunt for our dysfunctional penis.

What the Pennsylvania State College of Medicine list as putting the romance back is:

Re-acquainting yourself with your partner.

Openly discuss your feelings and concerns.

Discuss feelings about self-image.

Be patient.

What happened to dressing up, discussing your fantasies, going to a hotel and getting something lodged in your partner? That's romance.

It is at this point I realise what is disconcerting me about the presentation. It's the strange choice of images that have been used to help us understand the real issues being discussed. The next slide is on getting back your libido, which is helpfully represented by a kitten laying playfully on its back. I hope that's not helping anyone's libido. "Ooh kittens".

Sexual positions are discussed next, and whilst, more appropriately we have an image of the Kama Sutra, the look on the face of the man beside it suggests he's just drawn a big penis inside it. The subtitle reads "What is the best position for sex when having trouble breathing?" I would suggest if you are having trouble breathing you STOP! We all love sex, it great, but I put it second behind breathing on my most important activities.

Oral sex. Indeed. So what about it? Should having a transplant stop you enjoying "steak and blow job day"? Of course not. But diet is important as we are all told, so you may want to introduce "oily fish and blow job day" instead.

There are many images that spring to mind when someone mentions "oral sex", and for most of us it's picturing the last time we had it, or thinking of a lady happily munching away on a banana. For the Pennsylvania State College of Medicine, oral sex is best presented by the picture of a puppy with a children's dummy in its mouth! This is helped by listing the various fungi you can find down there. So, remembering that word "romance" again, you might want to gently whisper "it's alright love, I've washed it".

Eventually we move onto erectile dysfunction, and true to form we have a picture of the Leaning Tower of Pisa. I don't want to be over critical, but the Leaning Tower of

Pisa is still fairly erect in my book. It's pointing fairly skywards, and it's a fair old size. I'd be a happy man with that.

Advice is fairly limited about what you can do about this, ranging from counselling, vacuum devices, suppositories (ah, maybe that's how people get things lodged) and injections. Surely the key advice, and one that I would give any man going through this after transplant, is "don't worry, it's perfectly normal and common". Why is there no reassurance?

There seems to be two main problems here. First is that patients are naturally reluctant to discuss their sex lives openly, and secondly, the transplant clinics and national charities don't really want to discuss it either. The best we get is "Do you fancy it? Well it should be alright, please remember to breathe". Shouldn't we be more open and honest than this?

On my trawl through the web, I stumbled across this question listed on a general health website:

"My new boyfriend had a heart transplant 5 years ago and is doing wonderful. I would like to know if he can perform oral sex on me or is it something he shouldn't do because of his immune system?"

I'm sure this is more than fine, it's just a question of normal hygiene and knowing that you are free from any sexually transmitted diseases. But couldn't this be in the British Heart Foundations guide? Couldn't they mention how common problems are after transplant? That it is all generally fine?

So in order to help, and clearly as I think people shouldn't be afraid to say what issues they have, here are a few of mine since transplant.

Erectile dysfunction - on more than one occasion I have been let down by my own "Leaning Tower of Pisa". Worse when you are with someone new. I always think if they get upset by that then it's more their issue than mine. Generally if I worry, it gets worse, so best just enjoy what you can and it'll soon be back to "Straight Tower of Pisa" in no time.

Warts - lovely hey, but seemed to be a general side effect of one of my many drugs (I forget which one). I got a lot of them, and a man in a white coat took great delight at freezing them off. In fact I think he began freezing things that didn't even exist, such was my jolt at each shot he delivered. They eventually went, and were never deemed to be transferrable.

Boils - I've had these in my crotch and they were very painful I can assure you. My GP asked me if I would let a group of second year medical students look at my groin to see if they could spot the problem. My big fear of one of them saying "yes he has a small penis" proved unfounded. Thank you students.

Blood in my semen - this one shocked even me, but I happened to notice that my semen had come out a rather rouge colour. You don't imagine that's going to happen, and if you do maybe you need a new fantasy in your head. I'm on blood thinners so there is always a chance of a bleed and patently that's what had happened. It soon worked itself out.

So, if other transplant patients are experiencing something similar, then really the message here is "don't worry". Well maybe tell your GP, but only once you have finished the act itself.

But what about changes from pre-transplant to post-transplant? That's really what this book is about, and whilst the medication has obviously had an impact on my sex life post-transplant, has anything else really changed?

Most of the reported cases regarding cellular memory spoke about changes in sexual preference and also increased libido. It's quite difficult to remember what I was like in my pre-transplant days and whilst I could give my old partners a ring, I'm not sure it's a conversation they are going to particularly want.

I would say that my libido has increased since transplant, but I don't think that would be particularly unusual. After all, if you had been seriously ill for a number of years, then it's likely that would affect your appetite for sex. Subsequently, getting a new lease of life and getting well again is likely to increase that appetite. Only the drugs may push that drive down.

Oddly for me, I find my libido is at its highest when I am unwell. I'm not quite sure why that is? Either my body wants those endorphins to help give me a boost, or maybe it is something that is a distraction from the anxiety I get when feeling poorly. Either way, you generally are not at your most attractive when snot bubbles are coming out of your face, so it's not particularly helpful.

But does an increased libido prove anything about my donor? Not at all. It's so hard to judge, and whilst some people have had extremes in their drives and behaviour, I'd still put this down to the effects of ill-health and medication.

Changes in preference seem much clearer, and less explained by medication or other factors surrounding the transplant itself. Some of the recipients experienced a complete change including the sexuality of any prospective partner. Why would having a transplant make this change? Surely it must be the sexuality of the donor that is the major influencing factor?

Well it could be, but if you search any other number of serious illnesses such as cancer, strokes and epilepsy, you will find stories of patients experiencing changes in their sexual behaviour, including changing their sexual orientation. Operations, such as a transplant, are life changing and the stresses and drugs involved could, although very rarely, have big changes on your sex life.

So have my preferences changed? Well if you assume that the most extreme change anyone could undergo is a change in their sexuality, then no. I'm certainly not a homophobe, and I would have no problem if that was my sexual preference, but there has never been a hint of that.

There are other sexual preferences that are less extreme but still the sort of thing you would probably know about yourself. I'm sure if you suddenly gained an interest in bondage, then you have a rough hint that your preferences have changed. If unsure you could always ask your dominatrix what she thinks.

Other preferences are much more subtle. What type of person do you normally go for? Well I've dated blondes, redheads, brunettes, skinny girls, curvy girls, career motivated, family orientated and many others in between. So I'm not really sure what my preference for someone would be.

Equally, I've not really changed in the sort of activities I enjoy. It's remained fairly consistent despite the different partners. The only real change I could put my finger on is that I have a penchant for a nurse. Many men do I suspect, and when you have been put in the care of nurses much of your adult life then it is no real surprise you might find them attractive. Of course when you consider my libido is higher when ill, it does make a trip to A&E just that little bit more enjoyable.

I still need to fully test my sexual preference, and that's bound to be interesting, but as things stand I don't believe any change has taken place.

Having a transplant is a very intimate experience. You really are two bodies becoming one, and it is no surprise that some recipients feel intensely close to their donor. A report by Bunzel in 1994 on heart transplantation and sexuality had this to say on its closing comments.

"One patient confirmed that he was fantasising about the sexual habits of the unknown donor of his heart."

I'm sure most of us don't go that far when thinking of our donors, but the last comment is still as true today as it was in 1994, when I had my own transplant.

"It seems that physicians often neglect to talk about sexual matters with their heart transplant patients, though the patients consider it a very important topic."

Talk about it. And don't get anything lodged.

Test 5 - The Gay Test

"Susie's straight now. I mean it seriously. She was gay and now her new heart made her straight. She threw out all her books and stuff about gay politics and never talks about it anymore."

Brother of Suzie, a 29 year old heart transplant patient, and case number 5 in research by Paul Pearsall into cellular memory.

I'm confused. Or at least I think I am, despite being very sure of myself. I'm faced with a question that seems perfectly simple to answer, yet I'm unsure as to why it should be important or relevant to the answer I'm after. I've logged on to gay-test.com and it would seem I know little about what it means to be gay.

Of all the stories about character changes in transplant patients, it's the change of sexual behaviour, and in some cases sexual preference, that are the most dramatic. Could a donor heart really turn you gay? I very much doubt it, but it's something I should investigate. My donor may have been gay, and whilst I don't think my preferences have changed at all, maybe I'm not really looking for it.

My first step was to do some research into how someone would know they are gay in the first place. I'm not sure a quiz is the right way to find out, but I was hoping it might offer some clues. As a child I worried what would happen if I was gay, but it seemed the moment passed and I just naturally fell into chasing girls like many of my friends.

Back to the quiz and that strange first question "How much did I pay for my last haircut?" It was £21 to be exact but the options are in dollars, so I select the $25-$40 category. What about bald gay guys or indeed bald straight ones?

As I move through the 20 questions assessing my sexuality I start to wonder about what sort of person has written this. It seems strangely homophobic asking variously about my style choices or my preferences for musical theatre. I'm feeling like this doesn't have any particular research merit, but I press on regardless.

I finally finish what is a rather stereotypical list of questions and click on the button that says "get results". It states that I am 23% gay, giving the illusion of accuracy. The questions posed didn't indicate that any great precision would be possible.

Whilst this could suggest my heart is gay, yet I am not, I sense I need to delve a little deeper and see what real people go through when questioning a huge part of their make-up.

I go to the site for Stonewall, a charity and lobbying group that was set up to prevent attacks on gay, lesbian and bi-sexual people. Along with their campaigning of gay rights, they publish much of the latest research relating to gay issues.

I read through one article which discusses the question of whether a gay gene exists. It's an interesting point, as the genetic make-up of my heart is that of my donor, which is why my body tries to reject it, but if there was a gay gene wouldn't we be able to test for it?

The article reviews the various studies that have been carried out, including those on twins and suggests that although there is an indication that genetics may be a factor, environmental factors play a large part as well. As a race we are hugely advanced scientifically, but there is so much we really don't know.

As I read through I'm shocked to find out about how homosexuality was treated as a mental illness in the past. I always knew this fact but the real surprise came from the information that the World Health Organisation didn't officially declassify homosexuality as a mental illness until 1992. Are we really that slow in moving forward? I hope not.

I read through more and more information from various respectable websites such as the BBC and the NHS. None of them define how you would know you are gay, but simply suggest that it's a personal feeling and state of mind, and something that there is no reason to feel worried about. Fortunately I'm not worried, after all why should anyone worry about their sexual feelings?

This isn't going to be an easy test to judge, after all it's hard enough for some people to establish what their feelings really mean, and I'm somehow trying to assess if just my heart might be gay. The confusion in some transplant patients who have reported changes is striking, with one 25 year old male reporting that having a woman's heart has made him understand a woman's needs better.

"I never told anyone at first, but I thought having a woman's heart would make me gay. Since my surgery, I've been hornier than ever and women just seem to look even more erotic and sensual, so I thought I might have gotten internal transsexual surgery. My doctor told it was just my new energy and lease on life that made me feel that way, but I'm different. I know I'm different. I make love like I know exactly how the woman's body feels and responds almost as if it is my body. I have the same body, but I still think I've got a woman's way of thinking about sex now."

I have a male heart, and over the years I am pretty sure I have sussed out the workings of the male body too, like most men I've fiddled around with it enough. Maybe that's the difficult part, as a man receiving a man's heart, and of a similar age, maybe there isn't much to notice in terms of changes.

Many of the reported cases of cellular memory do seem to involve instances where the organ has been received from someone of the opposite gender, been much younger in age, or from a different racial background. Yet those transplant patients experiencing changes didn't know information about their donor until *after* reporting their changes in behaviour. Maybe we all have these changes, but it's only when the reality is put to us we make sure the narrative fits with our belief.

I plough on regardless, hoping that I will come across some information that will help me assess the sexuality of my heart. One website has a few more logical questions for me to think about.

Be clear on your definition of gay.

In the strictest sense I would define it as a man having sexual feelings for another man, but of course that could also include someone who is bi-sexual. Goodness it's a minefield, but if someone is gay then I guess that also precludes sexual feelings for the opposite sex. I spend far too much time thinking about the opposite sex, as many of my partners have complained about.

Understand a bit about what science says about being gay.

Obviously my initial research based on the "gay test" could not be classed in any way as "science", but the reports on Stonewall's site certainly helped. My problem is I'm questioning science as it is with cellular memory, so how much should I trust the science for homosexuality? Science always wants to define us down to a series of genetic markers, and whilst that helps eradicate disease, being gay is just an emotional state that I don't think can be categorised in that way.

Think about your past romantic experiences with the other sex.

Much easier and something that feels a lot more comfortable for me. The opposite sex. I note that it states "romantic experiences" and wonder how many of my encounters could be classed as that? Certainly the stripper in Benidorm was far from romantic, as most of the people in the room at the time would agree. Now I'm concerned I'm over compensating and trying to display my masculinity. Maybe, but I'm at least answering honestly. I carry on thinking for a while longer. No, no good. Just the stripper in my head now.

Think about romantic experiences or fantasies with the same sex.

Ah, now this is where it gets harder. Already I realise I've just typed a rather Freudian slip, but choose to ignore it all the same. I need to hear my heart as well as my head but no fantasies leap out. I fantasise about being a footballer and you don't get much more homo-erotic than goal celebrations, but I'm sure most boys dream those. I do have romantic notions about Sufjan Stevens, the American folk artist, who plays and sings with such quiet tenderness that I'd imagine he would make a great partner. Maybe that's my 23% coming out. Maybe the "gay test" was more scientific than I imagined.

Examine your recent behaviour with your friends and acquaintances.

The majority of my friends are female, and yes I can feel everyone reading this jumping to the same conclusion, but I just like female things. And football! Very much football. I have two very close male friends and yet there isn't much evidence to go on.

Sean, my music companion, sent me a text recently with four kisses at the end, and I immediately picked him up on it. One is fairly normal between us, but four? That's almost a relationship to me. He said he'd been texting his daughter and had just gone into auto pilot. Maybe Sean should take the test too.

My other male friend Yomi is good for a warming, comforting hug. Like being pulled into the clutches of a warm bear. He once hugged me whilst I was stuck in my chair in the office. I looked terrified, he looked delighted.

Examine who gets you aroused.

Do they mean actually examine, or just in my own mind? People often seem to ask you about which celebrities you fancy but I'm generally not very good with popular culture. Jennifer once spent a whole evening laughing at me because I asked about "Tiny Temperature". Apparently that's not his name.

I do my best to think of my favourite people. Nigella Lawson of course, full of dark thick hair and curves, and she can cook a bit too. Emilia Fox who plays Nikki Alexander in Silent Witness is another, mainly for her classical looks and stylish dress sense. Thinking about it, maybe it's the way she deconstructs a heart whilst performing an autopsy. No. Definitely the looks. Men? Well, as I mentioned before, I like Sufjan Stevens but I couldn't say that he gets me aroused at all, which is a shame as he is lovely.

So what has all this told me? Is there anything that leads me to think that my heart may have belonged to a gay man? Maybe I should read some books on the subject, but that's just going to throw my "Amazon recommends for you" list completely out, and I already get offered knitting books on the basis of my Christmas shopping two years ago.

To make any progress I really need to hang out where gay people do, try and mingle in and see how I feel. In this age of tolerance though, I would hope I already hang out where gay people do, because we are all just people going about our everyday lives. I don't have any particularly close friends that are gay, but that's just because I haven't made any effort in that direction. Friendships just happen naturally.

A couple of gay clubs exist locally, and that seems like a good bet, but I don't feel confident enough that it would be right. It has nothing to do with the "gay" element of it, I'm sure many straight people attend too. It's just the clubbing, and that's passed me by now. I've done my stint and I'd feel as out of place in a straight club as I would a gay one, and that won't help.

I have enough awareness to know that the local Gay Pride celebration usually happens around this time, each year. Maybe there will be something for me there? I go into the website for the organisation and download the programme of events. Much of it looks more ideal even if some of the events sound a little intense.

There is a "coming out workshop", which could help, but I imagine it deals with those young people that already know they are gay, lesbian or bisexual and are struggling to accept it. I'm not sure it would be fair to interrupt something so serious. There is singing with the local Pride choir. Again I'm not sure it will fit, after all a choir is a choir regardless of its combined sexuality.

I keep flicking through and a few pages in lies my opportunity to relax happily and comfortably, celebrating all that it means to be gay. What's more there is a picnic and entertainment thrown in. What more could a man want? Well possibly other men, but the Pride organisers have probably got that covered.

The one problem for me is that I should be volunteering on that day, helping adults with learning disabilities to cycle around a forest. Will I be able to fit both events in, without rushing my feelings too much?

The day arrives, and the cycling has already exhausted my energy reserves and delayed our arrival back in Norwich, but the opportunity to witness the Pride event up close is too great to miss. It's a short stroll down to the gardens where the party is in full swing, and as Jennifer and I make our way, I can sense a real feeling of nerves. I'm not sure why that is.

I often talk about the transplant family, or community, and how everyone really looks after each other. My sense is that the gay community is very much the same, and whilst that can be extremely helpful to those involved in it, maybe it also leaves those on the outside feeling more like strangers. It's not that I don't feel welcome at all, just not a true member of the club.

As we get closer the noise of party and celebration starts to fill the air. It has a real sense of occasion and joy to it, and whilst my nerves don't exactly settle, it not an intimidating place to be at all. This all feels new to me, and that's both in my own mind, and I think also for my donor.

The first thing that strikes you is just the sheer brightness of the event. The rainbow colours of the Pride organisers filtering into your eyes from every conceivable space and angle. Everyone is making an effort and so my main feeling now is not about belonging, but a feeling of being very underdressed.

The atmosphere is one of a carnival, friendly and jovial, and it's hard to not join in with that feeling. It's wonderful to see so many people together just celebrating sexuality, whatever that sexuality may be. In some ways, having just come from helping people with disabilities, it feels a shame there isn't an annual celebration of that too. A sense of community is so important, and that's what I'm really enjoying here, whilst still feeling a little bit of an outsider.

We spend our time just strolling around and taking in what is obviously the closing moments of the party. People are looking relaxed, happy and as though this has been something important and a day gone well.

I try and listen to my donor heart, but it's still nerves that are coming through and in many ways I feel a little guilty about that. Everything here is so welcoming and it makes no matter whether I am straight, bi-sexual or gay. Maybe I'd like to fit in more, but just don't know enough people to start. I feel more certain though, that this is a head and heart feeling, neither myself nor my donor truly belong to this club, but that's fine. Sexuality should be celebrated in all its forms and if my donor and I are both straight then that's wonderful too.

I head off with Jennifer as we discuss what we have seen, and look forward to getting a rest from our day's activities. Talk centres on how lovely it is to be in a city like Norwich where diversity is celebrated so positively. It makes me proud of my home city, and pride is the one word that stands out today. Norwich Pride, a celebration of the lesbian, gay, bisexual and transgender community, and one I was happy to be a part of.

Meeting Your Donor Family

"Those involved may want to exchange anonymous letters of thanks or good wishes through the transplant co-ordinator."

Advice on the NHS Organ Donation website for people wishing to register their organs.

In July 2009 an anonymous article appeared in the Guardian's life and style section under the intriguing title "I am following my birth father on Facebook". The author talks about finding her father almost by accident, the shock of that first look, and the near obsessional viewing of both his and his new daughter's timelines.

That was five years ago, and according to Facebook's own statistics in 2008 they had 100 million users, and as of today that's grown to 1.11 billion. Twitter was only launched in July 2006 and already boasts 645 million users. Social media is certainly big.

Where once we made sure that our phones numbers were ex-directory, today's generation would consider it extremely odd to want to make yourself anonymous. Get out there. Show the world who you are and what interests you.

When I had my transplant in 1994, social media certainly didn't exist, and the World Wide Web was only just coming into being, and not anything that was being used like it is today. The only way to contact your donor's family was via the transplant unit and vice versa, and all this was done anonymously too. You never knew who your letter was going to. Today those same rules apply, but the world is changing.

In December 2013, the Daily Mail ran a story about 21 year old Will Pope, a heart transplantee of just 12 months. Remarkably the story revolved around Will's meeting with his donor's father Steve Ince, who had first made contact with Will via Facebook.

On seeing the headline, so many questions filled my mind. Was Will ready for this kind of emotional exchange so soon? Did he even want to meet his donor's family? How had he felt receiving messages via Facebook? What did the Ince family want to gain from a meeting? Were they hoping that their son's spirit lived on within Will?

Those first 12 months after a transplant are a testing time, and anyone that has lost a child will be able to tell you that after only 12 months emotions are still highly charged. It feels like a risk meeting so early, but then again, what do I know?

Certainly Will had made the same connection between his donor's death and his own chance of life that I had made.

"I was aware that someone had to die for me to live, which was difficult to accept."

Difficult indeed, and maybe harder when the realities of that situation meet you face to face.

Steve Ince had read about Will's recovery from a heart transplant in a previous Daily Mail article. Putting two and two together, with the dates matching that of his son's death, he set about searching out Will on Facebook, finally mailing him with the message "I am the father of the donor of the heart you received."

Will was naturally surprised to receive the e-mail, but from his responses it seems he was genuinely touched by the contact and the opportunity to thank the family for their selflessness. It probably says a lot about the donor/recipient relationship that they both just wanted to express their feelings.

It appears that both parties had spoken to a psychologist prior to their eventual meeting, which was recorded by ITV. The words conveyed to each other are the same words you hear from all recipients. Words like "amazing" and "gift". There is also the sense of hope that donor families all must have "I feel like it couldn't have gone to a better person."

The immediate response from Will certainly suggested the meeting was valued.

"It was tough, but it was also cathartic at the same time, I don't know if we will meet in the future, but I am certainly open for any contact if that is what Steve and his family would like. I am so happy the meeting happened and feel much better for it, and I hope Steve and Sue feel the same way."

Will had been a fairly high profile patient whilst on the waiting list, his story appearing in national press and through television coverage. So could the same thing happen to other recipients, or was this just a one off?

A close friend of mine, Bec, is the mother of a 13 year old heart transplantee. Her daughter had a transplant back in 2002 when just 18 months of age, a mere 24 hours being the fine line between death or survival. On such slim margins does life hang, and when things work out you are going to be extremely grateful.

Over the years Bec has sent letters and photographs via the hospitals transplant co-ordinators. Like many the relationship has always maintained a certain distance due to the anonymity afforded by the process.

Although the donor family naturally wanted to write back. It had been a difficult process, until some 9 years later in 2011, a card arrived.

"I had just split up from Eloise's dad so presumed it was a "thinking of you" card from a friend. I opened it swiftly, it was a floral picture on the front with no words. I then started to read, I felt overcome with emotion and very upset, with no warning I had a reply from Eloise's donor's mum (R). I felt shaky but moved by the letter. It was lovely to hear that she thought of us often and donating her child's organs gave her great comfort. I always hoped that knowing Eloise was alive and living a good life helped ease just a tiny bit of her anguish and pain. That something positive came from her child's death. I treasure that card and showed many people."

More letters followed over the years as the two mothers continued a bonding process over the kind of emotional link that very few of us can ever experience or imagine. As I've mentioned before, transplantation isn't a cure, and isn't always easy, and in 2013, Eloise went through a period of rejection. Her body's immune system was trying to overcome the heart that she had lived with for nearly all her life.

"Once getting over the initial shock my thoughts turned to R, it seemed awful that Eloise's body was fighting the donor heart. I worried about R and would it be like reliving her daughter's death if something awful happened to Eloise as well. More heartache, pain, loss and grieving. Picking the scab off of a healing wound. I decided though that honesty was the answer and decided in my next letter I would explain what Eloise was going through, in an easy to understand way."

But before Bec could write that letter she spotted something unusual on her Twitter account. Both Bec and the donor mother were following the same charity, and with Twitters open nature it would mean that the donor family could read all Bec's tweets. All the hopes, fears and thoughts of a mother watching her child go through the roller coaster ride of rejection. What would you do? Bec had to widen the contact that maybe she wasn't quite ready for, certainly not in those moments of concern for Eloise.

"I felt quite sick and worried. I'd recently voiced concern that I was frightened of meeting the donor family and of them meeting Eloise. This brought with it feelings of guilt so many transplant families hear nothing from their donors and here I was saying actually I don't want to meet up. However I always said I would go with the donor family's wishes as I feel I owe them so much. I was also worried as at this point Eloise was experiencing her second bout of rejection. I decided Twitter wasn't the place for this to play out so I gave her my email address."

Luckily the two women continued to forge a strong relationship out of the love for both of their children. One fighting strong, the other never forgotten.

"Here was a mother who had experienced far worse than me, the death of her child and yet she thought of others and let her child become an organ donor. Strangely though emailing each other feels so right and so comfortable. We have probably shared more than others could ever comprehend."

All of us share our stories online. The need for more donors means we need to shout loudly about our success in order to help those still waiting on the list, ensuring they remain in the public consciousness. But in doing so, and by just sharing our daily lives and details on Facebook and Twitter, we could find our donor families looking in and seeing a story that might not always be positive. The fears, the depression, the struggle to cope. For Bec though the future looks positive.

"I know whatever battle is now sent my way I have someone I can rely on to support me, we're connected forever because of two amazing children. I think we will meet this year mother to mother, we are very similar woman, both with a nursing background. Together we can promote the Organ Donor Register, every story has two parts, I am just lucky to have the other half to Eloise's story in my life."

Both Will and Bec had the shock that social media can bring you in sudden contact with the family of a donor. But what if the meeting was set up as a surprise for you? We've all had the odd, surprise birthday party, people jumping out from behind doors, lights switched on, party poppers popped. Surely no-one meets their donor family like that?

Jim Gleason is a heart transplant patient from Philadelphia, who like me is an old time transplantee, having had his operation back on October 19th 1994. A proud person, Jim's the kind of man the transplant community rely on to promote just how positive the surgery can be. Like many patients, he attends his country's transplant games, showcasing just how normal life can become after a period of ill health, and providing thanks to the donors that got the athletes there in the first place.

During those US Transplant Games in Disneyworld, Florida a surprise was made for Jim to meet Gilberto, brother to Roberto, who was Jim's young donor. The meeting was set up to allow everyone to share the beautiful donor recognition ceremony that was part of those Games' events. Gil brought his partner, Luis, with him.

"Roberto has his roots in Brooklyn NYC and that is where he was attacked - on his birthday - on the street and beaten about the head with a baseball bat, lived in a coma for 9 days and declared dead October 18th 1994"

I find it hard to imagine how a family comes to terms with a violent, sudden death like that. In fact, it reminds me of the suddenness of all donor deaths, of families suddenly thrust into a world where they are asked to consider someone else's life. We say we would all donate, but in that position, what thoughts run through your head? It's obvious that Jim's donor family are brave people, and meeting definitely has mutual benefits.

"We had a very warm and welcome meeting, after the ceremony going out to dinner together. It was fun and very comfortable. We talked about how the decision came to be made along with some information about his brother's life and cause of death. Each year I write a thank you note (as I am doing today) to be delivered on our anniversary. He in turn shares it with the family (only brothers and sister since his parents pre-deceased him). On rare occasions we chat by phone as we did last night, but that's not anything regular."

Had knowing about the way that Roberto died affected the way Jim had coped with the transplant? Many of the stories involving cellular memory see patients reliving moments that seem reconstructed from their donor's death.

"No, not really. That was his life, and not mine. God is in charge, not me, so I don't feel connected beyond the story and no, never have had any flashbacks or dreams about the attack. I did eventually obtain a copy of the newspaper article describing the incident, no photos, written in Spanish - so I had a friend translate it for me."

Jim comes across as an inspirational figure to me, a man keen to give talks to groups about the positive impacts of organ donation, and always using the story of Roberto to bring alive the gratitude and bond that exists between donor and recipient. In chatting to him it became clear the transplant had given him a whole new confidence in front of an audience, and seemingly at ease with a large group of nurses. Was there something of Roberto in there?

"As for that talk today, the nurses laughed just as all classes do in response to that sharing about Roberto being a ladies man - and today, based on my call with Gil last night, I added that he was shy. About 70 in that class - good group - always well received, especially in contrast to the opening half hour of transplant/donation process facts presented by OPO staff - so mine is an easy and fun part of that time."

Jim is definitely his own man. After a near death experience I think we all find other aspects of life less intimidating. Not much can come close to the fear of those moments prior to an operation you know a big part of you is leaving. Jim has his own thoughts on cellular memory.

"I don't have any of Roberto's traits as best I can tell. He enjoyed his beer and a drink not so often, I never drink nor care for the taste of beer, either before or since this transplant. He loved baseball and football, while I enjoy a game every once a year or so, I don't follow sports at all, can't even tell you who's playing in a Super Bowl or World Series until the day of a game, even then, it's a maybe. He also loved collecting and wearing hats, gaining the nickname "Capone" for his often worn favourite 'gangster" type hat. I never wear a hat (except a huge sombrero one if out in the sun per my dermatologist's direction), so nothing passed along with that heart except a really healthy and strong beating one."

The photo of Roberto on Jim's website, shows a young, handsome, strong featured man. Resplendent in uniform and looking nervously, if not proudly out from in front of the flag of the United States. A picture that any mother would be proud to have on their mantelpiece, it's one Jim is very proud of too. I think Roberto would be proud of his recipient too, especially when in front of those nurses.

So what advice would Jim give a fellow transplantee who wanted to meet their donor family?

"With insights from many recipient/donor family communications in my network I would say it's a very individual thing."

As in the UK, the American system has intermediaries for each region (58 of them across the country, each independent with different levels of staff to support the process) and they facilitate letters which may or may not, over time, lead to names being shared and eventually on to a face-to-face meeting.

"I would say to write that letter - definitely - but how far to go beyond that anonymous letter writing, inviting direct open contact only if you feel the urge to do so."

Maybe Facebook and Twitter are opening up the world, our lives becoming more of an open book as we choose to share our inner most thoughts to strangers passing by the web. Maybe there is a danger we will be found through that process, and more donors and recipients will meet without the safety the hospitals look to provide. Maybe.

One thing the stories of Will, Bec and Jim has taught me is just how much we all just want to connect. A part of someone's family is now part of someone else's. Yes it's just an organ, but it's still part of someone. It's bringing life, and to that extent its life carries on.

I'm reminded of how hard that 10 year letter took to write. Agonising over it, trying to make sure it was right. I'm then also reminded that a family had to agonise over a decision very, very quickly and with a choice that could save lives.

The families make brave decisions, and yes it could be hard to meet, but I think the families deserve more.

Maybe it's time for a change.

The Case for the Opposition

"The idea that transplanting organs transfers the coding of life experiences is unimaginable."

Dr. John Schroeder, Stanford Medical Centre

Last month, a woman from Lancashire claimed her literary tastes changed radically following a kidney transplant. Cheryl Johnson used to enjoy celebrity biographies and best sellers such as 'The Da Vinci Code'. But now she prefers classics such as Jane Austen's Persuasion and Dostoevsky's Crime and Punishment.

Character changes in transplant recipients are known as cellular memory phenomenon. However, medical experts are sceptical about the concept and insist there is little convincing evidence.

As usual the Daily Mail provides yet another story that seems to provide further proof that cellular memory does exist. The Daily Mail seems to have a never-ending supply of these stories, and yet not much space is given to the scientific response to these claims apart from the final line "medical experts are sceptical about the concept and insist there is little convincing evidence."

So what do the medical experts have to say? Are they really that sceptical? The first question that surely needs answering is can an organ like a heart really store memories?

Professor Bruce Hood is the director of the Bristol Cognitive Development Centre at the University of Bristol and the author of 'SuperSense: Why We Believe in the

Unbelievable', 'The Self Illusion: How the Social Brain Creates Identity' and 'The Domesticated Brain'. Professor Hood has conducted a great deal of research into the brain and is clear on how memory is stored and the likelihood of memories being stored by other organs.

"Memories are encoded in the cerebral cortex and hippocampus and these brain areas cannot be transplanted. Nor is there any reputable evidence for storage of mental states outside of brain tissue. Organs are indeed connected to the brain via nerves but it is a totally different type of nerve system to that of the cortical neuronal networks of the brain that generate the mind."

If you are like me and not as clever as someone like Professor Hood, you may understand why we find it easier to believe a story about someone suddenly developing a liking for fried chicken. We understand it. We may not think it plausible but we can get the link. When we hear from scientists it's still hard to understand what they are really telling us, we either trust the boffins or we trust those that seem more like us.

In 2011, a group of researchers from MIT produced a report with the customer friendly title of "Optogenetic stimulation of a hippocampal engram activates fear memory recall"

In the report the researchers show how our memories are stored in specific brain cells. The scientists triggered a small cluster of neurons, allowing them to force a subject to recall a specific memory. When they then removed these neurons, the subject would lose that memory.

So if we accept that only the brain can store memories, and particular parts of the brain at that, then is there any other way that the memory could be passed to other organs? Rather than contain a specific memory, could an organ contain a sense of its hosts being? Could that "essence" just be absorbed by other ways other than just transplantation?

Dr John Schroeder is the Professor of Cardiovascular Medicine at Standford School of Medicine. He argues that the gaining power or strength from this kind of essence is a long held, but ultimately magical belief.

"The magical thinking of our ancestors may account for the first beliefs in something like cellular memory. Eating the heart of a courageous enemy killed in battle would give one strength. The practice of eating various animal organs associated with different virtues such as longevity or sexual prowess is one of the more common forms of magical thinking among our earliest ancestors. Even today, some people think that eating brains will make them smarter."

Dr Schroeder goes further to dismiss the notion that an organ transplant could somehow pass on memories to its new owner.

"If all cells are carrying information that can be passed on in transplant, why wouldn't this information be transferred when we eat fruits, vegetables, or any other living thing?"

It sounds a compelling argument, and none of us worry about the type of personality that our chicken breasts, minced beef or fish fingers may have contained. Maybe we should have new labelling "Aberdeen Angus beef, sunny disposition but not good in mornings".

But, to me, there is a subtle difference between eating an animal and getting an organ transplant. Nearly all the food we eat is dead tissue, it's no longer a living organism. Even food we swallow whilst it's still alive is quickly digested and seen off, so it doesn't remain living within our system. After all, we don't "reject" our food from our body. Well ok maybe after a rather eventful Saturday night, but not in the way the body tries to reject another living organ inside our body.

The belief that we can take on the essence of something living inside us, naturally feels stronger than the idea of just ingesting that essence. Margareta Sanner, a researcher in Sweden, has found that the general population fear that transplants using animal organs could lead to animal type behaviours in recipients.

"With regard to animal organs they reflected on the possibility of becoming more animal in their character, or beginning to grunt, or developing a snout."

Sanner was carrying out her study in order to understand what people thought about transplantation, and to help assess why donor numbers remained low. It seemed clear that there wouldn't be public acceptance of animal organs for transplant, but the fears of developing characteristics from the donor lessened when the donor was a human rather than an animal.

"For human organs the comments were more vague and usually concerned personality changes, above all if one were to receive a heart."

One of the most interesting aspects of Magareta Sanners report is the findings she made on the differences between recipients who received their organ from a deceased donor, and those that had a transplant using an organ donated from a living family member. Those patients receiving a kidney from a relative were not as worried about gaining personality traits from the donor, compared to those patients where the donor was deceased.

Sanners report provides statistical analysis of how comfortable the respondents are with each different type of transplant. The study indicated that 77% of the Swedish public were willing to accept an organ from a relative, 69% from a deceased person, 63% an artificial 'organ', and 40% an animal organ.

So the more different the donor, the more likely we are to fear that we will become like them. The research was carried out on those people not expecting to go through transplantation, and from my own experience the fear of gaining characteristics is overridden by the extreme fear that losing your life brings. Given the choice, most of us would just take what we can. I suspect afterwards that "fear" has turned into gratitude at whatever or whoever has saved your life. The sense of difference becomes something to embrace, a new essence, a new vitality.

This vitality though is sensed more clearly when the donor is again more different from ourselves; patients getting an organ from the opposite sex, older patients getting youthful organs, or a transplant from a donor of different race.

A further report called 'Another person's heart: magical and rational thinking in the psychological adaptation to heart transplantation' by the Shalvatah Psychiatric Centre in Israel, backs up these findings.

"46% of the recipients had fantasies about the donor's physical vigour and prowess, 40% expressed some guilt regarding the death of the donor, 34% entertained the possibility of acquiring qualities of the donor via the new heart. When asked to choose a most and a least preferred imagined donor, 49% constructed their choices according to prejudices, desires, or fears related to ethnic, racial or sexual traits attributed to the donor."

But what about changes in taste? Some of the desire for different foods is striking, and whilst it is easy to say you like a new style of music or feel a new vigour after your operation, a change in taste seems much more real and tangible.

Dr. Jeffrey Punch is a Professor of Surgery and Chief of the Section of Transplantation Surgery at the University of Michigan. He believes the simple reason for people developing new tastes is simply down to the powerful medication we all take to prevent rejection of our new organs.

"Side effects of transplant medications may make people feel weird and different from before the transplant. For example, prednisolone makes people hungry. The recipient of an organ transplant develops a love of pastry and finds out the person that donated their organ loved pastry as well. They think there is a connection, but really it is just the prednisolone making their body crave sweets."

I know just how much prednisolone makes you crave food from the amount I was eating following transplant. I'd had some extra large doses of the drug following a period where my heart had started to be rejected by my body. I found it impossible to stop eating, gained two stone, and had to avoid leaving any snacks anywhere in my house. A chap who had a transplant at the same time as me could almost order the entire menu from a Chinese takeaway and still get through it. I never did get to ask him if he liked Chinese food before his operation.

For the researchers and scientists who oppose the theory of cellular memory, it is obvious that memory is stored in certain areas of the brain and those other organs such as the heart and kidneys don't contain personality traits or an "essence". They suggest that we, as transplant patients, have just been through an emotional and physical journey and look for coincidences that then fit our donor profile.

For many transplantees it appears obvious that the donor's death had to come before their own survival and transplant thus making them feel proud and wanting to know their donors more. There is no other way for many transplantees to get an organ without the death of a donor and the two are naturally related. What it means is that many of us feel as though the two were linked, that the donor had to die for us to live, and that somehow we were in part responsible for their death.

You may find that ridiculous, but speak to anyone who has spent time dying, waiting on the transplant list. I'm sure every one of them has secretly hoped for a death to happen. I know I have. When Adrian was waiting on the list, the doctors reminded us that at the weekends more accidents occurred as youngsters partied. Would this weekend be that weekend? As you drove your car and someone stepped in front of your path, it felt like you could just go that bit faster, save your own brother. So when it happens, of course the natural feeling is that you're partly to blame.

Matthew Hutson author of 'The 7 Laws of Magical Thinking' and former news editor of the magazine "Psychology Today" explains this thinking as the theory of causation.

"We judge A causes B if A happens before B, A is consistent with B, and there are no other obvious causes of B. The trick is that this causation heuristic is so general that we don't distinguish between physical and mental causes. Event A could be an action or just a thought. If you picture something and then it happens, it's hard to fully dismiss your premeditation as an influence."

Causation also plays a part in my survival guilt with Adrian. Adrian's death revealed my own heart problems. Without his death, I would never have known about my health and probably died myself. In my head he saved me, just like any big brother would. The two don't need to be linked. We could have both survived. My survival wasn't a cause of his death.

With all this guilt and gratitude it's no wonder many transplant patients struggle with the emotional impact of it all. The Israeli report "Another person's heart: magical and rational thinking in the psychological adaptation to heart transplantation" concludes that the ongoing stresses involved are bound to impact on patients.

"Heart transplant involves a stressful course of events that produces an amplified sense of the precariousness of existence. Simultaneously, it gives rise to rejoicing at having been granted a new lease on life and a clear sense of new priorities, especially with regard to relationships. Less expectedly, this study shows that, despite sophisticated knowledge of anatomy and physiology, almost half the heart recipients had an overt or covert notion of potentially acquiring some of the donor's personality characteristics along with the heart. The concomitance of the magical and the logical is not uncommon in many areas of human existence, and is probably enhanced by the symbolic nature of the heart, and maybe, also, by the persistent stress that requires an ongoing, emotionally intense, adaptation process."

For those with a more scientific knowledge of medicine and the workings of the human body, cellular memory simply does not exist. The fact that there are any number of stories out there with transplant patients gaining new and interesting tastes or desires, does not make cellular memory any more likely. Dr Schroeder believes we are just attempting to pull together such stories to help fortify our belief.

"Collecting stories to validate a hypothesis is a risky business. Stories of transplant recipients that don't seem to exhibit memories from their donor don't prove that they aren't there, but those stories are selected out anyway. Stories that do seem to exhibit donor memories don't prove cellular memory but collecting a bunch of them could lead one to see a pattern that isn't really there."

I'm aware that's very much what I am doing, but does it cause any harm to see if cellular memory exists, even if it is fairly unscientific. For many there are genuine reasons to be concerned. The earlier Swedish research highlighted that people are more concerned with donating theirs or their loved ones organs if they think their personality traits could be taken on by a patient. Stories like the one in the Daily Mail could easily have a negative impact on donor numbers, just as it could through my own writing. That's a concern for me, but in reality I know the numbers reading this are like to be handfuls rather than thousands so any impact is minimal. I understand that fear, but part of me thinks the more we get the discussion out in the open, the more we can ask and deal with the reasons patients feel this way. It's because of a love for their donors, and that should be positively promoted.

Maybe it's time for the scientists to look further into cellular memory, but as Dr Schroeder states it needs to be done thoroughly.

"Science should be moving us forward, bringing about a better understanding of how phenomena work. Scientists like Gary Schwartz and Paul Pearsall introduce mysticism and magical thinking into the mix, which is very attractive to many New Age healers because it supports their spiritual leanings. However, such thinking does not advance science; it takes it back to an earlier time, a time when the world was dominated by magical powers."

For many though the trouble with science is that it baffles us with its explanations and theories. Science needs explaining in simpler terms to us, and because we rarely get offered answers in those terms, it seems like a closed shop. New age theories then offer alternatives we can understand and fill the gap. Science doesn't need to be more open, but it just needs to show it still accepts that we don't understand everything. For Dr Schroeder the stories from transplant patients shouldn't be dismissed out of hand.

"An organ transplant is a life-altering experience, literally. In many cases, it might well be compared to the near-death experience since many transplants are done only if death is imminent. It should not be surprising to find that many transplant recipients change significantly. Even so, the stories are intriguing and may lead to some serious scientific investigation at some time in the future."

One question I hear often from transplant patients is "How do the doctors know how we feel when they've never experienced an organ transplant for themselves?" It's a good question and something science can't really answer. Those of us that have gone through the trauma of the operation know what an emotional experience it is. For Professor Bruce Hood it's an example where the practical is harder to understand than the theory.

"I am not sure how I would react to someone else's organs inside me. On an intellectual level I know that organs are just component parts that serve a function but to be honest, I think I too would have to fight hard not to believe that I had part of someone else living on inside of me. It's only natural."

Test 6 - A New Love

"We made a great joke of the contract but he still agreed to sign, I just hope it will save his life."

Martin Warburton (a Manchester United fan who agreed to give his brother a life-saving cell transplant on the condition that his sibling sign a contract stopping him supporting arch-rival Manchester City.)

I'm city 'till I die,
I'm city 'till I die,
I know I am,
I'm sure I am,
I'm city 'till I die.

It's a chant every football fan knows, and sung with gusto, changing the "city" to the relevant part of their football clubs name.

It suggests that once you have chosen your team, there is no room for change. It's forever. It's not like a marriage or a best friend, this decision is unbending and unbreakable. "I'm city 'till I die."

As chants go though, it does have some weaknesses. Firstly, if I "know I am", then really there is no need for the next line in the chant. I know, end of discussion. Yet we get the element of self-doubt that creeps in with "I'm sure I am". So maybe a need to double check in the mirror.

There is also the "city 'till I die". Football has long been compared to religion, yet for all fans it seems there is no room for reincarnation or the afterlife. For them, supporting their chosen team stops at death. Surely we should be cheering on the boys for all eternity?

Despite this I have always been "city 'till I die" and Norwich City to be more precise. I chose the team of my birth, the yellow and green "canaries", and became a season ticket holder aged 12 and never looked back.

So how much of a fan of my beloved canaries am I?

My teacher at primary school had to speak to my mother about my habit of only colouring pictures in yellow or green.

My bedroom walls were also yellow and green with the picture of every player adorning them.

I was a ball boy for two years, mixing with the players and generally handing them back things they thought they had lost.

I cried when we won the League Cup at Wembley, and even more when we got relegated. I've travelled to different countries just to see them play.

So I know I am, I'm pretty sure I am, I'm City 'till I die. But what about this heart? After all that only became part of me in 1994, and what was its allegiances before then? City? Rovers? United?.... Town?

I still had the scientists rejection's of cellular memory in my head, but I still had the ultimate test yet to come, that of love. Love can move in very mysterious ways, and for

Connor Rabinowitz of Minneapolis a heart transplant was to lead to an unusual matching.

Post-operative and recovering well, Connor wrote a letter to the family of his donor, Kellen. The reply was equally swift, leading to a meeting with Kellen's mother Nancy and his sister Erin, within 12 short months.

"It was an emotional meeting and as Nancy put her hand on my chest to feel Kellen's heart beating inside me, I saw Erin for the first time. We locked eyes – and I was smitten. Erin felt the connection too but she tried to dismiss it, thinking I was too young."

After a few years out of contact with each other, Connor and Erin got back in touch via Facebook in 2010. It seems the connection between the pair was too strong, and after a long distance relationship, the couple finally moved to be together.

"All of the family tell me stories about Kellen. He is always in my thoughts – and obviously in my heart. He was a great guy – he always looked out for people. Through him, I hope I can do the same. If I was to meet him today, it would be like meeting my other half."

Maybe the donated heart really does know who it loves, and if it does then wouldn't I feel that love too?

I'd thought a great deal about how I could test the concept of love, toying with the idea of multiple dates and even going so far as to try my own harem of different, potential partners. As nice as the plan was, it did seem rather time consuming and maybe hung on my ability to find enough dates to assess who my donor might like. Just finding one had sometimes proved elusive, so failure looked certain.

There was one love though that had remained throughout my life, and that was of my chosen football club, so seeing if I could love another could be the test I needed. It would be highly unlikely that my donor was a Norwich fan, but with the majority of men having a passion for football the chances are high that my donor supported and loved another team.

What if that team was Ipswich Town? Would I be able to celebrate a goal scored by my local rivals? Would I feel my donor heart leap as the ball hit the back of the net? In his book "The Self Illusion" psychologist Professor Bruce Hood asks if you would accept the heart of a murderer if you needed a transplant. Many wouldn't. I'm also sure the same number of Norwich fans would say they wouldn't accept the heart of an Ipswich Town supporter, but maybe, just maybe, that's what has happened to me.

The rivalry between Norwich and Ipswich is an intense one, and one that is separated by a county border and forty miles of flat farming land. The hatred is deep and fanned by the local press and also the teams themselves. My own badge of honour came at a visit to my local GP, an Ipswich supporter since birth, yet he still does his best to keep me healthy. He managed to spill one of my urine samples over himself, leaving me gleeful in the fact I had now pissed on a member of the self-called "tractor boys". He didn't look quite as happy.

Working in Norwich, you do find that the odd Ipswich fan has had to migrate to the bright lights of Norfolk in order to find employment. You'd imagine they would want to keep themselves hidden away, but this persecuted minority does tend to make its voice heard. Generally they appear the moment Norwich City suffers a defeat, joyfully stomping on any remaining positivity that may have come out of a game. So when I needed a ticket, there were already a few people I could speak to. The question was, dare I ask?

The truth is, I had been putting this test off for a while. Out of all of them, it's the one I panicked about most. Football has been a life long passion and even visiting Ipswich seems a very strange idea to me. Illogical but still strange.

With the season quickly running out I needed to make a move, so one lunchtime I started browsing eBay. Now, normally when a colleague shouts "Oh my God, what are you doing?" it would suggest your computer has some horrendous or morally indecent image on it. In this case it was. I was viewing an Ipswich Town shirt, and I was looking to buy.

A debate quickly ensued, and I was left in no doubt that any change to my allegiance would mean losing the respect of those that work with me. I couldn't show my face, I was going to become an outcast. Support soon arrived though, and the resident Ipswich fan dragged her knuckles along the floor and made her way over (for the record her knuckles are regulation size and don't touch the carpet).

The opportunity of "turning" me was not one she was going to miss, and as luck would have it she could get me two very reasonably priced tickets for their forthcoming fixture against Derby County. The offer was now there. If my donor was an Ipswich fan, this would be the only way I'd find out.

There seemed to be multiple benefits to someone else buying the tickets. Firstly the ticket office wouldn't ask difficult questions about my Norwich address. Secondly, it felt like I wasn't putting my own money directly into their coffers, and lastly, I wouldn't get on the Ipswich mailing list and find myself shamed every time I opened the door to my postman.

Tickets organised, I went back to my eBay session. Shirts, all blue, none of them appealing, but I needed to select one. Did it matter? I could just burn it afterwards in some kind of cleansing ritual. Just look for the cheapest I thought, and with that as my selection criteria I bought a 2007 home shirt for the princely sum of £7.25 (including postage). I would say it was a bargain, but it felt extremely overpriced.

A date was now in my diary, I felt as nervous as I had ever been in a long time. No one cheats on the love of their life without feelings of guilt and shame. The longest relationship of my life was heading for an examination, one that could ruin the one thing that keeps me going.

A few days later and my eBay purchase was swiftly with me. There is normally an element of joy to be had in trying on a new item of clothing, especially in adulthood where it's less likely to have been a knitted gift from an elderly relative. Today that new item is in the blue and white pinstripes of Ipswich Town, and holding it out in front of me, it might as well be an orange jumpsuit from Guantanamo Bay.

Looking around, despite the relative security of my apartment, I pull it over my head and try to sense if any part of me is enjoying or feeling comfortable in this moment. Nothing. Dare I look in the mirror? It's like that moment when you know the haircut you requested was wrong, but until you see it for yourself you can kid yourself it hasn't happened. It has. It did. I looked like an Ipswich fan, albeit a very anxious and unhappy one. In many ways I fitted in.

Match day is normally an exciting moment for a football fan. Full of hope regardless of how previous results have been. There's the joy in seeing familiar surroundings, lush turf, tribal colours and sounds. I was going to be heading into the unknown, a wolf in sheep's clothing (or rather a canary in a Suffolk Punches garb), an imposter, a double agent.

The plan for the day was to head off to work, get changed straight after, meet my friend Sean for a bite to eat and then jump on the train to Ipswich. All simple, but from the moment I changed into my new identity I felt worried about anyone seeing me. Walking into a local pub in Norwich dressed in blue and white is not advisable at the best of times. Try explaining to the landlord that you're just testing to see if your donated heart came from Ipswich. I'm either going to be beaten up or institutionalised.

Fortunately by the time we arrive at Norwich station, there are one or two exiled Ipswich fans waiting to get the train, huddling together for safety. I smile nervously. No one smiles back. There must be some kind of secret sign. Sean busies himself with ensuring we are getting the right train. I'm just assuming these blue clad football fans are going our way.

The closer we get to Ipswich, the more I become less of a stranger, but part of a blue family filling out the carriages with the excited chatter of promotion prospects. It's a warm and familiar feeling, but I feel unable to join in for fear of exposing my true colours.

The train finally pulls into Ipswich Station. At this point in any journey, many Norwich fans will take the opportunity to use the train's toilets, hoping to flush their excrement over the tracks, marking their territory. Could I? Should I? I was still thinking like a "canary", and I wasn't making an attempt to listen to my heart. I needed to connect somehow. But how? Walking along from the station I felt a thousand eyes upon me, each questioning my being and piercing through my blue and white disguise and into my soul. Did they know?

Normally on my walk to Norwich's ground at Carrow Road, I'm filled with excitement and questions about who will be in the days line up. This walk is different though, I realise I hardly know any of the Ipswich players, let alone who I think should be playing. As for excitement, it was still just nerves, a worry of being discovered in a hostile environment. We need to look as though we know where we are going. To stride out with purpose and familiarity.

Fortunately the first part of the ground that we come to is the Sir Alf Ramsey Stand, where Seán and I will be located at the front of the top tier. This is an area marked for "home fans only". I smile slightly too much at the assistant on the gate, hold my ticket out, and breathe a big sigh of relief as the turnstile clunks me through. I'm in!

Whenever you go to a friend's house, it's never quite as nice as your own, and Portman Road is no different. It feels like the bar areas could use a freshen-up, and nothing under the stand seems to shout out about glories past.

We make our way up the stairs towards the top tier. On my way I see lots of signs for the local brewery "Adnams". I like their beer. I like it a lot. Now the drink feels a little tarnished. A bitter taste will be added to my bitter from now on.

We turn through the entrance to get our first glimpse of the pitch, and make our way through a throng of supporters all looking to get to their seats before kick-off. Ours, at the front of the stand, are easy to find, and I soon find myself looking over the edge and down to the blue and white sea of colour below. My heart quickens, but I'm now just thinking about the game ahead of me. I want kick-off to arrive.

The referee blows his whistle to start the game, and the majority of the 17,000 strong crowd are in their seats and ready for 90 minutes of action. The small few yet to be seated seem to be heading my way, and apart from late they are extremely drunk and boisterous. I stand to let this rough looking group pass me, as they shout at people to get out of the way.

Suddenly there is large roar from the away section of fans. We are only 34 seconds into the game, and Derby has scored. My first taste of real action as an Ipswich fan and I missed it because of the lout in front of me. The goal was apparently turned in by Patrick Bamford, after a cross from the left. Even those listening on the radio will have a better idea of what happened than I do. Bugger.

Finally everyone is in their seats, but I feel slightly disconcerted that the drunken, hooligan element has chosen to sit right behind me. If my heart really is an Ipswich one, it needs to convince me and my new friends breathing down my neck. The pressure really feels on.

Playing today for Derby is former Norwich striker Chris Martin, a local lad who had both supported and played for the yellow and green. I had been expecting some ritual abuse of him from the crowd, but they seem slightly ambivalent about his presence. That soon changes as Martin snaps into a challenge on an Ipswich defender and appears to push him in the face for good measure. Cries of "scum, scum, scum," are aimed in Martins direction, and from behind me, just to confirm to everyone else the enormity of the situation, I hear "He's a Norwich player, get 'im off!" That's cleared that up then.

Things start to heat up as Ipswich try to force their way back in the game, and as challenges start to fly there comes a loud chant from behind me of "Who are ya? Who are ya?" I feel fairly sure it's aimed at the Derby fans, but it's very clear who "they are". Could they mean me? Are they questioning my authenticity as an Ipswich fan? I try to join in the chant but nothing falls from my lips. I undo my jacket so more blue is revealed and try to relax.

The first half proves to be a frustrating affair, with a lot of pressing by the Ipswich players but without actually forcing the Derby keeper into making a save. The half time whistle blows and as yet I feel my performance as an Ipswich fan measures that of the team. A lot of effort but not enough pride in the shirt.

During the break the discussion behind me starts to take a more odd yet sinister tone.

"I'm fucked," slurs one drunken voice.

"You're fucked," responds a voice in a tone not far removed from a psychopath that's just been stung by a wasp.

"I'm not fucked," the slurred voice counters his own original statement.

"You are fucked," the psychopath clarifies. At least he is sticking to the script.

"Yeah, I'm fucked," the drunk and equally confused voice finally confirms what the rest of the people around him already know.

Then the conversation turns darker and slightly more troubling for my worried mind.

"I'm going to push him, I'm going to fucking do it," states our confused drunk.

Push who? Me? I'm right at the edge of the upper tier. Surely even a drunken idiot wouldn't be so stupid.

"I'm going to fucking push him over."

So it's "over" now. He does mean that someone is going over the edge, and who better than the cowardly Norwich fan and his crap disguise.

Staring in front of me, full of fear, I know what I need to do, and it isn't to jump before I get pushed. I stand up, turn around and pretend to be looking for some long lost relative at the back of the stand. Trying not to draw attention to myself I glance slowly down in the hope of understanding if it's me that is being talked about. I catch the eye of the psychopath. Shaven headed, battle hardened and in his late forties, he rises with purpose and embraces me in what can only be described as a headlock.

"What do you reckon?"

It's seems more questioning than inquisitive and tinged with the slight air of menace. I try and think of some Ipswich players to help me seem like a true fan, but none are coming to mind. I'm staring blankly, any longer and I'm bound to be discovered for what I really am. My donor really needs to talk to me now, but nothing is entering my conscious. I take a breath in, look my new friend straight in the eye and say "I think we're fucked."

I'm never sure that a smiling psychopath is any better than a scowling one, but for now it feels like a small success.

"That Williams lad is playing fucking well. We'll be alright yet" suggests my now calmer match analyser.

It's the "we'll" that comforts me most, even whilst his arm pulls ever tighter round my head. I have looked my enemy in the eye, and fooled him of my loyalty. Maybe this heart is Ipswich and closer to my donor family than I suspect. My head hopes not.

The players return, and once more we are in our seats and I'm starting to want Ipswich to win this game. I'm willing them on, if not being able to shout out any support. The match starts to turn the way of the "blues" and after 68 minutes, my psychopath friend is justified in his beliefs when Williams scores a spectacular equaliser. I cheer. It's a half cheer, but it is a cheer. It feels forced, but I'm going with the flow.

The action continues and Ipswich look the most likely to score, but time seems to be against them. Despite their best efforts it's seems the result is going to a draw as the game closes down into injury time.

Everyone is starting to shuffle towards the exits when Ipswich are granted a corner. The ball gets floated in and Aaron Cresswell meets it fully to send the ball into the Derby net. Ipswich have won the game and the blue family are all hugging in joyous rapture. Seán and I just stare, with a disbelieving smile, unable to fully join in the celebrations. The final whistle gets blown and "I feel like singing the blues" is played loudly over the stadium speakers.

It's a party atmosphere as we make our way out of Portman Road. The talk is all about the possibility of promotion and how much Ipswich are the team in form. Inside I can feel how much I don't want them to have success, but I still feel happy in the fact that this test is now through, and maybe that happiness stems from what I know to be true.

I'm city 'til I die.

Who Is My Donor?

"Maybe it is worth investigating the unknown, if only because the very feeling of not knowing is a painful one."

Krzysztof Kieślowski (Polish film director and screenwriter)

I'm struggling to breathe. I'm sucking in oxygen but it doesn't seem to be doing anything to the functioning of my brain, which feels like it's spinning round like an out of control washing machine. I stand up. The room joins in with the motion of my brain. The world is turning at a speed my body can't comprehend. I reach for a glass, fumble for the tap, and gulp in some cold water.

"Fucking idiot" I say to myself. Frustration turns quickly to emotion, and I can feel tears trying to force their way up through my sockets. I don't want to cry, I'm still angry with myself and unsure about what I've just seen.

My "tests" have been completed, and as each one has passed I've grown ever more curious about the donor heart that resides inside me, and the person whose life ended when mine begun. I've wanted to know more. In fact I need to know more.

I've written about heroes and villains. I've accepted that my donor might not have been someone I liked. They may have held completely different views to my own. They could have had a different culture and ethnicity. They could have been gay or even like Ipswich. What I do know is that they are a part of me. And I want to know that part more. To connect fully with this heart. To love. To grieve.

My head starts to clear a little. I put the kettle on for a cup of tea. The sound of the water starting to boil, soothing my mind as I take a few minutes just to wait and watch.

A few minutes earlier I'd done something I thought I had done many times over. I'd tapped in a little information about my transplant into Google and expected the usual vague responses. This time though, the first search item returned hit me full in the ribcage, sucking the oxygen straight out of me.

I still hadn't clicked on the link. Should I? Am I opening a Pandora's box? It still might be nothing, just some rogue coincidences that when seen in a calmer light will just reveal itself as a bland news story that has no effect on my life. I can go back to beautiful ignorance.

There are moments in life where you are faced with a choice. Sometimes it's as simple as the route that you decide to take home, but it can end up having a massive effect on your life. Do I take my usual route home tonight and leave this information where it should be, or do I take this new road, click the link and see where it leads?

I gaze at the scribbled list of characteristics that I believe my donor had. Looking through all the tests I've made it seemed to me fairly clear.

Test 1 (Eiffel Tower) - Donor feeling high, think they like heights.

Test 2 (Snowboarding) - Donor feeling low, though sense they like trying new things.

Test 3 (Accordion) - Donor feeling low, again sense they like trying new things.

Test 4 (Boyz II Men & rhubarb yogurt) Donor feeling high, definitely likes "End of the Road".

Test 5 (Gay test) - Donor feeling low, definitely not gay, but no feeling of prejudice either.

Test 6 (Ipswich) - Donor feeling low, definitely not an Ipswich fan, though might be a fan of another team.

Guess Who? Test - Donor is white, smart, possibly in a middle class profession.

Tea made and I put the list away. I sit back on my sofa. Never has one page of Google been stared at so intently. It's almost as if I want to see through those first lines and into the article without going into it. For good or bad, I'm going to look. I can't turn myself back.

What have I learned about my donor already? All I really know is age and sex, and from my list, I have some internal perceptions about the kind of person he was. It's like the person you only hear on the phone. I have built up a picture around little details, and after my tests I have formed that into a fully-fledged human I can see and sense.

They are 32. They are male. These are facts.

I see them as being physically active. Maybe not heavily involved in sport, but someone who has a body that hasn't as yet been slowed by a sedentary life.

My climb up the Eiffel Tower and my snowboarding sessions were situations where I felt my heart was ruling my head. I had fear, but there was a desire to go further than I had before, something was overwriting my thought patterns. I didn't know if it was my donor, but if cellular memory exists then it would make sense that my donor was less fearful than myself. I certainly get a sense of someone with a confident, fearless manner.

I don't think music plays a big part in their life, although I'm fairly sure that R&B is something that they listened to and enjoyed. There is something to that moment with Boyz II Men that goes a lot deeper than a memory of a song. I don't think the song is necessarily that important, but the band and the genre of music is something that has a strong connection.

That brings me to race. On my list I picked the white guy in the Guess Who game, and it's a question that I still don't feel I've fully answered. I have always pictured a white man, but I have a lot of doubt. I've come back to it time and time again and I wonder why. I really struggle to say for certain what I think. My head goes for white I think because it's natural to think of your own reflection when searching for yourself. It is a very tough call though.

They are the same sexual orientation as myself. Nothing has ever changed in my mind or my heart about my preferences. I certainly have a "type", but I know that hasn't altered but only strengthened as time has gone on. My failings may suggest I've never settled when with a female, but I'm fairly certain I'd fail with men too. I struggle with my habits, I don't need another me.

Food preferences are a difficult one to call out. There was nothing at all in rhubarb yogurt, and I can't think of any foods that I've suddenly liked. My tastes have changed over the years. My favourite food is curry, it used to be sausage casserole. I can't say what my donor likes. Sadly, nothing comes through that strongly.

So. 32 year old white male. Slim, strong and energetic. Straight, single and with a preference for R&B music. Full of life, a life sadly ended.

That's what I believe.

The facts remain that all I have is a 32 year old male.

No going back. I touch the link to the news article that's caused me so much panic already. It references the two facts I already know to be true. The death relates to a 32 year old male. There is also a name. A name. It's real, it's suddenly a person, a life. I can't describe how different that feels. I've felt the presence of someone unknown half my life, every heartbeat coming from another human I love and can feel. Now with a name it's as though I can reach out and touch them.

Then there are the other facts. The death. A violent death at the hands of others. I won't share the details on here as it's not fair to anyone, regardless if this person is my donor or not. It shocked me though, I had to read the sentence again and again, wanting to be sick and force out the pain coming from my stomach.

A name. Reality. And now that reality has a brutal ending that scares me. I'm wondering why it happened. I'm trying to put myself in their shoes, the family's shoes. My head is spinning again. It's like an overload of emotions and I can't find a fixed point to cling to.

Through the process of the book I've thought about many things to do with my donor, but oddly I'd never considered their death. I've never wondered how it happened. For some reason I'd always assumed it was a car or motorbike accident, and in time maybe that just became my accepted reality. This was something much more though.

A million questions started filling my head. The most important ones being some verification of the facts. Could this person actually be my donor? After all there must be hundreds of deaths on any given day, so the chances of a coincidence must be high.

According to the data 1,300 people die every day in the UK. The vast majority of these are through illness and old age, so unlikely to be suitable for organ donation. But around 45 people die each day from some form of accident, be it a transport incident, a fall or quite commonly accidental poisoning. Murders are considerably less common with around two murders occurring every day.

So prior to my transplant there could have been 40 to 50 deaths that involved either accident or murder. Potentially they would have been evenly split between males and females, making 25 deaths that would fit with my donor's gender. Spread that across the age range and you wouldn't expect more than one or two deaths for a male aged 32.

Donation could have come from death through illness, but again I wouldn't expect numbers to be high, although my level of knowledge in this field is limited. All in all it suggests a high likelihood that the person mentioned may well be my donor. The fact remains though that it is only likely, it is by no means definite and I could easily have stumbled across a coincidence.

Equally I worry about the nature of the death. Could they really have been suitable for organ donation? How quickly would someone make that decision? I understand that people died often from head injuries and that whilst brain dead, their bodies were still functioning through life support at hospital. I hadn't really considered death by other injuries. What was possible?

A lot of thoughts were swimming around in my head. I was desperately looking for some kind of confirmation, yet part of me didn't want to believe it was true either. The book was an intention to delve a little deeper into who my donor might be, and potentially get a chance to hear from my donor family about who this person really was. It was a slow, soft landing into the safety net of closure that the knowledge would bring. This was like being fired from a cannonball headlong into a brick wall of confusion.

I tried to rationalise things in my head. I had been foolish in looking, but what I had found was just a possibility. No more. I needed to calm down and chat to someone about it. I needed perspective.

The question of who to call wasn't a problem. Jennifer and I had gone through a lot of difficulties that had ultimately ended in our separation, but she is still the person I trust the most. The person that knows what makes me fearful. The person that knows how to be calm in any given situation.

"I've done something silly" I said down the phone. I'm unclear why we play these guessing games when we speak to people and "something silly" could be a multitude of things.

"Don't worry", came the assured reply. "What is it? Are you ok?"

"I think I've found my donor."

Sounding confused and unsure if she had heard me correctly, Jennifer started to sound more concerned.

"What do you mean?"

"I was writing my book, and thought I'd see how easy it was to find out information about my donor, so I Googled some stuff, and, well, I think I found him."

Soon Jennifer was going round the facts in the same way I had been the previous half an hour. Couldn't it just be a coincidence? What about the dates? Can you remember being told any more about it when you had your operation?

It was good to chat, and I certainly felt a lot calmer speaking to Jennifer than I had been with my own muddled thoughts. The question though was what should I do next? Now I have some information how on earth do I verify it?

As I've mentioned before, donation works through strict confidentiality rules, and all transplant hospitals abide by these thoroughly. Even if I was to ask my transplant clinic to confirm or deny the name that I now have, they are not going to. I want to ask them, but equally I feel very foolish. I feel like I've done something wrong, and like a bad child I'll be sent to my room and told not to return until I can stick to the rules.

Maybe the psychiatrist can help me through these questions? Maybe, but I'm fairly certain she already sees me as too intense following my last visit, and now she will only think I'm turning into some kind of soul searching lunatic. A casually dressed lunatic at that. I can't leave it here though. Too much of my life has been spent wondering, and I can't turn away when the answer seems so tantalisingly close.

There is only one thing for it, and it means doing that simple thing that I found so difficult ten years ago. I need to write to my donor family, I have to reach out to these amazing people I do not even know.

I have too much respect for my donor family, or indeed any donor family, to try and contact them through any other method than the correct channels. They don't need to meet, or even respond, but I would like to know more about the person that first owned this heart of mine.

It takes a few weeks before my head can deal with the shock of discovering a name. I keep running it over in my mind and I discuss it with a very limited number of close friends. It's clear there is going to be a lot of doubt around my donor's identity so it's not something I want to talk about in my letter. All I'm really asking is to know more.

Now to find a card. I hate this part. Where do you start when trying to find a card that reflects outwardly by its picture, how you feel. Flowers? Blue skies? Sunshine? None of these really do it for me. For help I look back at the card I received from my donor family all those years back. It's a blue card, with a strip down the middle showing Egyptian Hieroglyphics and various pyramids. I can't imagine picking this myself, but did I care when I received it? I don't think I even looked, it was all about the words. Maybe I just shouldn't worry so much. I find a simple card with red butterflies flying out of a field of bamboo. Thank you Paperchase.

My first mistake is to start writing out my feelings directly onto the card. First of all I haven't fully considered what I need to say, and all that comes out is a flurry of emotive words trying to express a gratitude that sounds, well oddly, half-hearted. Secondly I have made that very schoolboy error of only leaving an inch of white space for my closing paragraph. My text size is shrinking with every poorly written word. I finish, ashamed and upset with myself.

I think the problem here is the desire to say what I think my donor family want to hear, rather than what I actually want to say. I'm trying too hard to make them aware of my gratitude, when that should come through naturally if I just be myself.

I've still got a couple of weeks before I'm due for my check-up at Papworth, and that's the time I will have to hand over the card. With that deadline in mind, I decide to just wait until the words come to me and sketch them out on my phone first. Hopefully then I'll come up with something decent to say. Most of all I need to ask more about my donor; I need something real, and this might be my only chance of truly finding out.

Days pass, and I'm still swirling thoughts around my head about the information from Google. I go back and forth to the article I found, but in a calmer, more considered frame of mind. I don't want this knowledge feeding into my donor letter, yet it feels hard to ask a question when you think you know half the answer. Time is ticking on and I'm no closer to having the words I want.

Pressure is building now. My appointment is only weeks away and I'm having to spend today in London on work's business. Nothing has been written, not even outlined. I'm tired, I'm on a train full of commuters but I need to start getting something down. I look out the window as the world seems to race by, I daydream for a minute about my life, and return to a blank screen. The first word is typed onto my phone, then the second and before I know it I have a flow going on. It feels right, and it feels like this is what I want to say. Within 20 minutes I have my draft, and it also feels like it's the final version. Happy and relieved I relax into the last half hour of my journey and start to think about my day ahead. Phew.

It's always hard looking back over words when they are finally written in black on a stark white page, but I will always feel I couldn't have written anything better. I'm sure there are some amazingly moving donor letters out there, and I'd love to see more of them, but here is mine.

20 years is a long time. For me it's time I thought I'd never get, for you the passing of time must still be a painful reminder of the loss you suffered.

I've always understood that I could only survive through the bravery of others, of a decision to end a loved one's life and allow others the opportunity of life that organ donation brings.

20 years ago I was a 23 year old boy, frightened that my life would be over before it began. I'd lost my brother on the transplant list, his battle too short. My mother was looking at losing us both. Your decision changed all that, and the grief I felt for my brother extended to this unknown, incredible donor.

For 20 years your son's memory has been as big a part of my life as my brother's. I think about them both every day, luckily I can look at my brothers picture, see memories, shared moments, love. But for this other person that is such a major part of who I am. I have nothing. No image, no knowledge, an unknown donor who I feel such gratitude and thanks for.

Time has passed and it may be a chapter you have, or want closed, but if you feel able I would love to know more or see a picture of your son, my donor. He gave me life, and I have lived it, I now just want to be able to say a proper 'thank you'.

With much love. Mark.

The Longest Night

"84 infants died with 45 (54%) identified as potential donors"

The report 'The potential for neonatal organ donation in a children's hospital' by Great Ormond Street Hospital concludes that over half of the babies who died in neonatal and paediatric intensive care units could have been potential organ donors.

It feels such a weird point in the night. It's now 11:05, and I'm up in bed drinking whiskey. Fairly normal you would think, although maybe drinking whiskey in bed alone isn't on the NHS recommended list.

Tonight though I need it. Selfishly I've been thinking about how scared I feel, when a little boy is about to be taken down to the operating theatre for the miracle that is a transplantation. I can hardly breathe as I type, yet how on earth must a parent feel, a mother, watching her child disappear through those doors.

I think of my mother. Brave, scared, petrified even. And she did it twice. Well the wait at least. I only gave her scones and a pot plant for Mother's Day. Bugger.

11:19 and my messages have gone silent from Willow, the mother of little Theo, who is probably unaware of the amount of people holding him tight in their thoughts. Willow has been chatty these last few hours. A mixture of excitement, anxiety, panic and even laughter to hide the fear.

Another 3 minutes and nothing. Texts had been every few seconds, now I'm staring into the void that is a blank iPhone screen. Modern life, watching pixels and hoping they burst into life and indicate that the world is still moving in a positive fashion.

Again I'm thinking of me. Why doesn't she text? What's happening? Is Theo in theatre now? Silence surely means that worst moment is upon her, the moment of letting your child go into the skilled arms of another. To be opened up. The heartbeat you listened to when just an unborn child is to be removed and replaced with another.

Thoughts of the donated heart fill my mind. That heart too was listened to by an excited, expectant mother. She too is losing that heart. She had to let her child go for good, and yet in this moment she is allowing Theo an opportunity. I'm still completely amazed by the beauty of that.

My part in this drama, my very small part, my role of friend, has ceased for now. There is nothing more that I can do apart from wait. Should I read? Sleep? Eat a biscuit? Drink another whiskey?

My mind has gone blank. It's as if time is running through porridge. I know this is silly, and as much as I've got to know Willow and Theo, they are hardly life-long friends. Why does it matter so much? The emotional bond that transplantees feel for each other is a strong one, and stronger for those that still wait. I prefer to stay on the outside and avoid these moments. On the inside there is nothing I can do accept care too much.

Again. Selfish.

23:45 A message! A photo even. A little boy, for all the world looking like he is relaxing on the beach, eyes hiding from the full force of the sun, arms stretched behind his head as a makeshift pillow. If it wasn't for the tube from his stomach, the tell tale red wristband ensuring that you are the right child, then it would seem a happy pose. The next picture more unsettling. A scared looking little boy being comforted by his mother. My scared little boy emerges from my inner self, takes a gulp of whiskey and runs for the comfort of the duvet.

Oh my lord. Tears again. My brother would be so ashamed of me. It's ok, I'm alone. Just as a falling tree makes no sound, a crying man sheds no water. I do really need to do something else.

More messages have now been passed. I'm sure I should be offering words of advice, comforting phrases about how it's all going to go so well. In actual fact I'm mentioning all sorts from willies through to amusing chocolate bars (finger of fudge struck a wrong note). It's a distraction I hope, and for now the messages coming back suggest that it's a help of some sort.

00:25 and my kettle has been boiled and a cup of Horlicks made. Malty goodness for a twilight hour. I must be extremely old. It wasn't too many years back when a kebab stuck to the side of my face at 4am was the order of the day. Now I can hardly get through a small child's transplant without assistance from a warm beverage. Anyone in their right mind would have had a red bull and coke. Schoolboy error.

Peace descends again. 1:10. Time to put my light out.

The night drifts into a blur of fitful sleep and barely conscious messages at random intervals. My mind, unsure of the space around it, moves between my brother, my operation, Theo and sometimes just odd moments of terror. As morning arrives I make a cup of tea and imagine that everything will be done and we can start the emotional round of congratulations. As it is Theo is still very much unconscious and still not closed up. I can't imagine how someone so small is still managing to find strength after such an ordeal, but he's hanging on in there. That's all anyone can hope for.

In the brief chats I have with Willow, we both express our amazement at the strength of a donor family, but naturally Willow's focus is still caught in a huge mix of gratitude and fear for the immediate future of her son. How do you cope with all that?

My own thoughts about my donor hit me a good while after my own operation, so for now I'm trying to imagine what last night must have been like for another family somewhere? What did they go through? How were their emotions?

To help me I turn to a blog that had been written by one of my friends from Twitter. Sally had lost her son Toby following a slip from some cliffs. A sudden tragedy, unexpected and throwing life into turmoil. Yet in those tragic moments Sally and her husband had the courage to think of others, just like Theo's donor family last night.

Sally describes vividly how quickly one family's lives can change.

"We were enjoying our first day on holiday in Cornwall, a beautiful place called Cadgewith Cove. Toby slipped whilst climbing on rocks, from what we have been told he would have known nothing. He broke nothing, which I still find unbelievable, but the blow to his head was catastrophic. However, thanks to the quick thinking of three very dear people Toby was kept going long enough for the air sea rescue to get him to hospital and CT scans to establish brain death."

Right now Willow is fighting for her child. We've spoken before about when you can let go and know the fight isn't one that's going to be won. Can a mother truly let go of her son? It's only natural that you'd refuse to accept your child won't recover. I saw that with my brother. There was acceptance from some, but not from others. For Sally it says much for the immediate care of Toby, and the family's bravery that they were accepting of the clinical analysis of the hospital staff.

"Those first few hours are now a blur and I think I am probably glad they are. We were prepared for the worst by the first consultant we saw who told us that it looked grim, when Toby went up to ICU we were told that Toby was brain dead from the impact of the fall. It really matters that the consultant telling us cried as she did so. It left no doubt and gave us complete trust, we knew that they cared and would have saved Toby if they could."

When Adrian died it left me completely numb. I expected it, but it was still as though my mind didn't want to process the information. The following days were spent doing almost normal tasks, yet I can barely remember what I was doing at all. It was a fog. I couldn't think about anyone else. In fact I could hardly think at all, so how would a family manage to take their nightmare, and try and step into the shoes of someone like Willow? Many of us think briefly about organ donation when we are asked to join the register, but how many discuss it? It seems Toby was one thoughtful individual who did. An example to many of us.

"A couple of years ago Toby's grandma died, her death prompted us to have discussions about what we would want when we died, of course I thought it was me telling Toby my wishes, I am glad I did not know then just how important that conversation was to be. I remember saying to the hospital staff, you are going to ask about organ donation aren't you, the answer is yes. I remember how taken aback they were at how easy the decision was. But you see I remembered that conversation with Toby, we were sat in the kitchen and he said very clearly he would want his organs donated. This was therefore his final wish and the last one we could grant."

Many of us don't have that discussion and it can mean that a family overrides, quite naturally, the unknown wishes of their loved ones. Organs that could be transplanted never used. It's something we need to keep promoting. For many the rejection is not about organ donation itself. You've just lost someone very close to you, and the last thing you want is that person having organs removed and taken away from you. Sally's description of her final night with Toby is in extreme contrast to the rush of adrenalin Willow first felt when news came to her of a possible organ.

"Toby was declared dead at 6.55pm. The transplant team did not come for his organs until 10am the following morning. That was my longest night. Do you know how rhythmical a life support machine is? All through that night I listened to it, I stroked Toby's hands and face, I kissed him, I told him how much I loved him. We made painted hand prints, red for Liverpool. It was the hardest night ever, I never wanted it to end but I also needed it to end. I could actually feel my heart gradually breaking. We had to answer loads of questions, all so important in ensuring the best match, there were decisions we had to make that I never thought I would have to. The moral dilemmas you face, all with lots of support and all considering us as well as the potential recipients. Staff worked around us with such respect, keeping Toby's body safe until the transplant team could get there. They gave us such support, it made us strong enough to get through that night and make Toby's wishes come true."

For one family this is the moment when everything begins. New hope and the potential for life are whirring into motion. The chance you have been longing for all these months and sometimes years is upon you. For another it's the end of hope. Finality. Pain. Grief. Could you imagine what it would be like to be in the shoes of Toby's family?

"Leaving Toby was the worst thing I have ever done in my life, I knew that I would never see him again warm and soft and kissable.

"We had such a long drive home, but gosh did we smile when the transplant ambulance drove past us blues and twos going strong. That was my boy going to save the lives of others."

Saving the lives of others. Saving someone like Theo, who is now fighting all he can to make sure a family's gift becomes the most precious one he will ever receive.

"Just before Toby's funeral we had a letter to tell us the difference Toby had made, he had given his heart, his liver, both kidneys and his pancreas. Four families lives were turned around by Toby, they were given back life.

"I still hear it you know, Toby's heart, it has a soft gentle rhythm. Its a good heart, its strong and kind. I hope it gives a long and happy life to the recipient.

"When your child dies so does a big part of you, if Toby had needed a transplant, I would have wanted some other parent or family to make the same decisions that we did, it has given us some comfort and made us very proud."

I hope Sally and the rest of Toby's family know just how proud they really should be. Every transplantee is certainly proud of Toby and of them.

Weeks passed and very slowly Theo began to make the long journey from operation, to intensive care and finally back to his old bed at Great Ormond Street Hospital. The Theo that was before slowly started to return, and with that Willow began her journey back to mother rather than carer.

During those weeks something had struck me from talking to a few transplant families, something I'd not really considered before on this moral journey into cellular memory. It was prompted from the fact that Willow had photographed and subsequently kept Theo's failing heart. Many found it a little odd, but to me it had its own symbolic beauty. Most suggested they were glad the old heart had been consigned to history, broken, diseased, a symbol of the pain, fear and suffering they had been through. But why then did a donor family feel so different?

Cellular memory suggests we may carry around some of the thoughts, feelings and memories of our donors. Families meeting up with heart transplant patients have wanted to put their hand on the recipient's chest, to connect, feel the beat of a lost loved one. But if cellular memory exists what does that mean about the organs we discard. Why don't we feel love and grief for these organs? I've gained a new heart, but I've lost a part of me.

The insinuation is that my new heart is good. It saved my life, it was powerful, vibrant and strong. My old heart was weak, failing and going to kill me. I've never really given any thought to my old heart in the last 20 years, yet I've spent every day thanking and feeling the positivity of my new one. Each beat a reminder of another chance at life.

Yet our old hearts are a piece of history as much as Toby's heart is to Sally's family. Toby's strong heart gave new life, our old hearts sustained life long enough for that chance to arrive. We should feel proud and remember how much a huge part of our life it was.

As Willow shows me the picture of Theo's heart, all brightly coloured, a vivid blood red, fresh from the chest of its former owner, it looks strangely underwhelming. Willow appears more fascinated by its appearance, trying to almost look beyond the muscle and tissue to see what secrets it holds.

We laugh and joke about how strange we must look as we discuss a rather unique picture of a child's heart. It's difficult to know what a stranger might think should they stumble across the image, but it makes for an enjoyable debate.

So here we are, sitting, eating and chatting about that night again. A night when so much changed for two families. A night where fate entwines your lives in this strange, unique bond.

Theo has a new heart, it's letting him move from his hospital cocoon and back to the life with his mother and siblings. I wish Toby could be back with his family too, but the reality is that will never happen. To see Theo's face excited as he plays with his brothers, you know the amazing kindness of strangers means at least one life has hope and a future.

I look back at Theo's old heart. I feel only warmth and love. I hope Willow feels that too.

Appointment with Destiny

"Every day I try to picture your face and imagine what you look like. I think of you surrounded by your loving family - maybe your wife and children who miss you very much"

Hannah Jones who made headlines in 2008 when she refused a transplant aged 13. Now 19, Hannah has been transplanted for five years.

6:45 and the alarm goes off. I'm shattered. I got home last night at 11:00 after a business and social trip to London, so I could really use a rest, but today is clinic day, my six monthly appointment at Papworth Hospital to check on the state of my heart.

Maybe it's my anxiety, but everything feels rushed this morning. Maybe it's the emotion from little Theo's own transplant still effecting me. My hands shake as I grab and try and sort out my medication. I need to remember not to take my rejection medicine as I'll be having a blood test later to check on my general levels. The hot water from the kettle sloshes over the side of my mug as my attempt at making a tea suffers from my general lack of alertness.

I don't normally get too worried about these occasions, after all any routine becomes just that, routine. The anxiety is present mainly because I have my card for my donor family, and because it's something I should chat through with my consultant. In all my years going to Papworth, my donor isn't really a subject I've brought up, and so my routine is being disturbed by this emotional bump on an otherwise smooth road. Adding to it is the fact I'm still unsure if I know who my donor is or not. Today I could find out for sure.

7:40 and I'm picking up Jennifer, who is looking after me for the day, despite our separation. I never go to clinics alone, mainly because of some strange superstition that I have. When I was told I needed my new heart I was alone at clinic for the first time, so I've made sure I'm never alone again. Jennifer knows this, and her presence is a very reassuring factor.

.

The journey takes 90 minutes, through 75 miles of the Norfolk and Cambridge countryside. Time is passed by chatting through my latest plans to own a camper van, and we stay away from anything too deep and meaningful. Jennifer knows I'm anxious and doesn't add to it with questions about how I'm feeling.

We soon arrive at Papworth Hospital itself, a small, specialist hospital with an eclectic range of small buildings, portacabins, old cottage style units and modern concrete blocks. It's not pretty, and it feels a mess, but it's loved, cosy and to the transplant patients it's home.

I arrive at clinic at 9:40 and check in at reception. I should then hand in my blue book, something that the transplant patients record all their daily medication in. I've stopped doing this, mainly as it just felt like an extra reminder of a daily chore. I'm passed a blank sheet and asked to write down the drugs I take. To be clear, this isn't because the hospital has somehow forgotten, or doesn't keep records of all my medication themselves, it's solely to see if us patients are actually taking what we should be. You'll be surprised how easy it is to be taking the wrong dose of something.

First up is my bloods and a few little tubes that need filling. When I was a child this would have sent me into a screaming fit, with everyone around left in no doubt about the fear of a small needle. These days it's no different than brushing my teeth. Soon done and I'm off to get my chest x-rayed, something so simple you don't even need to take your top off for. In many ways it's underwhelming.

X-ray completed and I'm back to the clinic and Jennifer tells me she has a treat for me. This sounds exciting and I wait eagerly as she rummages around in her oversized handbag. It's a Finger Of Fudge. Now, I like those, but I can sense 30 pairs of eyes on me as I take the small confectionary item in my hand and stare at wonder at this little offering. I look up. Faces full of sympathy are looking at this man child, who sadly needs a reward for being well behaved during his blood test. A manly cough exits my throat. I rather aggressively hand it back to Jennifer and make her put it away. "Do you want it later?" she whispers. "Yes please" I reply, sounding again like the little boy I really am.

The room is extremely busy today, with no space to be had on the many blue cushioned chairs that fill the small atrium like space. When I first had my transplant the numbers seemed much less, and it felt like everyone knew each other, a family atmosphere was always present. It still has that, but I don't know anyone here. I feel like the distant cousin at a wedding party, a sense of belonging yet in some senses a stranger to all those around me.

I'm soon called through for my ECG, a process that involves being wired up to a little machine to record the electrical activity of the heart. It's painless and easy, but modern science, despite its giant leaps forward, has yet to invent little pads that can stick a wire to a hairy human being. Over the years I've had sticky pads, suckers, chest shaves, tape and quite a lot of improvisation. Today it's the latest version of the sticky pad. I keep as still as I can. The pads remain stuck. Now they just need to come off again, why anyone chooses to be waxed for hair removal is beyond me. I smile as they are pulled off, and wonder if Jennifer might have a packet of football stickers for me if I don't cry.

I'm no sooner out than I'm called by the nurse, a quick chance to check how fat I've become over the last six months and to do a quick test of my blood pressure. I normally find that my blood pressure rises on these appointment days, and probably due to the nature of visiting a place where Adrian died. Today it's fine, maybe after 20 years the place is beginning to lose it's demons for me.

I mention to the nurse my letter for my donor family, and she enquires if I have ever written before. I feel slightly embarrassed about the fact the last one was 10 years ago and I'm only now getting round to writing again, but we talk about my letters and how it didn't seem to me like the family wanted repeated contact.

The conversation progresses and then I'm faced with a question I'm unsure how to answer. "What do you know about your donor?"

Should I admit what I have found via google? Shall I say a name and see what response I get? Instead I play the game of bluff and say the facts which I'm sure of, age and sex.

The nurse smiles warmly "do you want to know more?"

"What do you have?" I quickly respond, half in excitement and half ready in the knowledge that I'm not going to get the answer I really want.

"We can tell you what the cause of death was"

My eyes are lighting up at this moment, after all this will be everything I need to confirm or deny my suspicions. If the cause matches what I have found then I can be fairly positive that I've found my donor. The nurse says she'll arrange it, and I head back full of nervous excitement to the waiting room.

I tell Jennifer the news, and she seems as surprised as me. I wanted to get some kind of confirmation about what I think I know, but didn't know how to broach the subject. Now I have, I feel like I've taken a giant leap forward. I'm starting to relax.

Before coming today I'd asked if I could see the psychiatrist lady again, so I could talk over my frustrations with the mental help I had been offered since I last spoke to her. I'm called through to a small room and this time I bring Jennifer through with me, mainly as I want to make sure I'm clear on how I've been feeling and she can help me facilitate that.

I make a little mental note that the psychiatrist is more casually dressed than our last meeting, but I don't bring this up, feeling that humour at this stage may detract from my real frustrations. I'm struggling. Badly. Sometimes it feels like you are shouting for help in an empty forest with no one listening. Taking Jennifer in proved the right decision as she airs forcefully what I'm really thinking. Finally it feels like I've been heard.

When my old heart was broken, every medical option and resource was provided to help fix things. My mind is a little broken right now, yet it feels like I need to work hard to get the help I need. Options are provided today, and that truly makes a huge difference.

Back in the waiting room and the mood between me and Jennifer is much lighter, with laughter as we joke about the amount of forms I'm being asked to fill out today. The mood doesn't even change when we are told we are last on the list to be seen today. Whatever went on in the room with the psychiatrist, it had a good effect. For now at least.

The room slowly starts to become a scene less full of anxious faces and one of empty, uniform chairs. The day so far has been one of positivity so I'm not worrying at all about my final appointment of the day, with one of the transplant consultants. Today I will be seeing Dr Clive Lewis, a relatively young doctor who I feel very confident and comfortable with.

Dr Lewis has that unique ability to make every patient seem like the most important person on his case load. Maybe "unique" is a bit strong, as it's actually an attribute that is shared by Dr Jayan Parameshwar, without whom I very much doubt I would still be here. I'm sure I am just another patient to both of these clever chaps, but they make it feel very different to that. Patients often remark about how amazing Papworth Hospital is, but a hospital is just bricks, mortar and technical equipment. It's people that make a place special and unique, and in Jayan and Clive we are lucky to have two great members of a brilliant team.

I walk in to the consultation room and as usual I seem a little confused about where to sit. Next to the table? Over by the examination bed? Clive appears to gesture towards some seats, so like an obliging patient I sit down and Jennifer takes the chair next to me. Finally a nurse uses the one spare seat and we are all in position.

Clive starts with the opening gambit of "how's it going?" I always feel at this point as though we're playing poker here, I share my information before the consultant shares with me how I should probably be feeling. The other problem with this initial question is the very English way we have of dealing with things in front of respected professionals. I've been in emotional turmoil and feeling like death the last six months so naturally I respond with a "not too bad, thanks."

I can see Jennifer looking as though I should really offer up a bit more than this meagre response, so I start to talk through my general tiredness, my anxiety issues, the fears I have for my future. Clive listens intently, and as usual he is being pushed into counsellor mode rather than cardiologist. The subtle difference is that Clive uses all his knowledge of my current health issues to help me understand we are far from being at the end of the road. He understands. We talk about how my heart looks, we discuss future possibilities. Now relaxed I again mention my card, and also my book.

"What's it about?" asks Clive. I hesitate. I want to say but also not to look foolish in front of someone who I trust my life to.

"Cellular memory, and how some recipients think they take on characteristics of their donors." I reply, waiting to be marched off the premises.

Clive responds with interest and is far from dismissive about the subject, instead acknowledging that there are many things we still don't know. As we discuss what I have done so far I find myself relaxing, handing over the card for my donor family and again saying how much I want to know more about the original owner of my heart. Clive turns to the nurse and asks if she has shared the details of what they hold on their own database, and we go over our previous conversation from earlier in the morning.

"Let's get those now" Clive says cheerily. And with that everything is set in motion. We close up our own conversation and confirm another appointment for six months time. I'm told to return to the waiting room and that the nurse will come back with the information I'm so desperate for.

The waiting room now only has me and Jennifer in it, but there is an electric tension in the room as I sit and imagine what I will be told, the consequences, the knowing. After nearly 20 years, the next five minutes could tell me the answer to a question that's been in my head nearly every day since transplantation.

The nurse calls me through, and I go in alone (on later reading, Jennifer told me she actually went in with me, but I have no recollection of this). She is holding a sheet of paper and it feels like time has slowed to such a pace we are trapped in a vacuum. I'm eager, needing to just get to the facts. I want to just know the cause of death. That's all I need. Nothing else.

I'm asked what details I know. This feels like the kind of repeated information that Chris Tarrant goes through on "Who Wants To Be A Millionaire" before revealing that you're going home with nothing.

"Well I know they were male and that they were 32" I state, sure of my facts and trying to cut to the chase.

"They were actually 31 at the time of death" responds the nurse, matter of factly, as if the minor difference makes no real difference, and why should it?

Time freezes completely and my head spins, and I'm not hearing anything the nurse is saying now. 31? How could this be? How could I have got it wrong? My heart sinks and I start to take in that the story I have found, the potential donor, they are no more connected to me than the coincidence of dying the day before my life was saved.

We don't even need to move to the cause of death, my hopes have been shattered, but as I regain a little composure I hear the details that are being read out to me. My donor died through a head trauma, probably through an accident of some sort. It's what I initially imagined happened all those years ago, but I can't get out of my head that I got the age wrong. I know one thing, cellular memory has a lot to answer for if it's giving me wrong details.

It feels less like a step back and more of a giant leap backwards into the unknown, both in getting to know my donor and also in the quest to find out if cellular memory really could exist. I'm crest fallen as I go back out to tell Jennifer what I have just found out. It feels like it might be the end of a journey, but one that has ended just as I was beginning to feel a real sense of belonging and closeness to my donor.

As we chat though, it's that very point that makes me positive again. I'd wanted desperately for my information to be validated, to allow the information to bring a name to this heart, to give me someone to cry and grieve for. I'd wanted that. That feeling was still there, if anything it had confirmed that I should be trying to get more information. That I could cope with knowing.

All had not been lost, I still had the letter that was now to be passed onto my donor family. For all my searching the answer now laid firmly and only in my donor families hands. 20 years ago, my life was in their hands as they wrestled with the decision to donate or not. Now all this time later, only they could answer my questions.

A wonderful family saved me once, it's a little unfair to ask them for more, but a little more is what I need.

Meeting the Family

"When I moved to embrace her, I could feel her thin and solid body grieving in my arms as we cried together. I felt a bond between us, a bond like nothing I had ever known."

Claire Sylvia on meeting her donor Tim's mother Mrs Lasalle.

Thursday morning, mid-July. Sunlight streams through my open window waking me far too early and making me grouchy already. My stomach doesn't feel much better and so I stumble down my stairs in search of tea and sustenance.

It's been 15 months since I started my journey. 15 months that have felt more traumatic than I could ever imagine, and has impacted heavily on my life in a myriad of ways. Now though, on this beautiful summer's morning it's going to come to its conclusion. It's a big day in a life of many big days.

My face is swollen and the heat has left me feeling exhausted, and to be honest I'm already feeling like this is something I don't want to do, but it's too late to pull out now. I also need to get the closure that Claire Sylvia's daughter Amara spoke about. Eating doesn't settle my stomach but the tea fares a little better.

Finally up and showered, I find myself distracted and unable to focus on one task at a time. Everything feels jumbled and my mind a fog. It's obvious I'm stalling for time. I'm extremely nervous and unsure of myself. It puts me in mind of all those times waiting pre-operation. It's the hottest day of the year and I spend a good 15 minutes trying to work out what to wear. In the end I plump for comfort and pick a dusky red polo shirt and green shorts. Unable to put it off any longer I make my way to my car.

En route I stop off at a Waitrose to see if I can find some suitable flowers and a nice plant or two. The supermarket seems a haven of slow moving, middle-class pensioners as I scan the brightly flowered stand. Unusually for a man, I like buying flowers but I feel a bit overwhelmed today, and choosing feels like the hardest thing in the world. In the end I go for the easy option and purchase two rose plants and a bunch of roses and carnations.

It isn't long before I'm finally at my destination, I pull up outside an old flint stoned wall, birds happily singing in the morning sun. My stomach churns over again, and my head pounds as a sickness tries to overcome me. Passers-by offer a cheery "Hello" to each other as I try and get myself out of my car. Why is everyone calm, when I'm in a whirlwind of emotions?

I take one of the rose plants, the one with yellow flowers and make my way up a long gravel drive. The whole place is peaceful with just the hum of traffic in the background and the sound of the odd wood-pigeon filling the air.

A few paces in and I can see the rows and rows of old gravestones as I make my approach. Large solid stones covered in various states of lime and moss, with one, a monument rising almost ten feet out of the ground. I turn to my right and walk a few paces across the grass and start to feel my heart heave and my eyes struggle to keep moisture at bay.

Flowers already surround the small cross that sits above the small square stone in the ground. I move some of the wilting flowers to the side and reveal a small plaque.

"Adrian P Watson died 13 February 1990 aged 22 years. At rest"

It's my brother's grave and one I haven't visited in a long time. The pain of doing so, far too difficult, having always felt more a vision of my future than some comforting place from the past. I gently rest my flowers down and take a deep breath. It's a part of my life that's always with me, just like my donor.

Adrian was a donor too, and whilst only his corneas could be used, that gift will have been just as large a one to a recipient as my heart is to mine.

I settle down beside Adrian's grave for a moment's thought. As I do, an old man with the whitest head of hair comes strolling past. "Communicating," he calls over. "Something like that," I respond with a warming smile as my nerves settle.

It's been nearly two months since my letter to my donor family and as yet, I've had no response. Naturally I felt saddened and disappointed but my expectations were always low. I just hope they got my letter. Through my writing, though, I'd realised that I had been looking at how much my donor had changed me as a person, how much their genes had mingled into my own. The truth though, is that my life had been shaped by my family, by my brother Adrian. And it still shapes it today, always hoping that he would be proud of me. As much as I needed to meet my donor family, I needed to reconnect with my own. Today I was doing just that.

Laying in the grass, something changed. This place started to lose a little of its fear and become something a little brighter. Maybe it was the sunshine, maybe it was just nerves easing. Whatever it was, my heart and mind felt at one.

Across from my brother's grave lie the smaller rows of stones for those children that have been lost far too young in life. The grass is more lush and the buttercups seem to know just where to flower.

The graves full of fresh flowers revealing that memories are hard to let go. I wonder how many of these children may have been donors and therefore saved a life like Willow and Bec's children? It maybe doesn't matter who my donor is, we all owe a lot of love and respect to anyone who has been through donation. Even if you've just added your name to the donor register you have my admiration.

I get myself up and take a last look at Adrian's small but heavily flowered grave. I will be back. I'm not sure when but I will. My next stop however, is one that is a little trickier. My father's resting place. Why tricky? For one, I have never been there, and second, because until recently, I didn't know he had been laid to rest at all.

Families can be difficult things, but they make us who we are, obviously more so than donors. My relationship with my father had become strained after separating from my mother, but I'd reconciled with him prior to his death from a brain tumour. His new wife had decided to keep his ashes, and although we didn't get on, I understood her reasoning. That's the way it remained, or at least so I thought.

One of my close friends, Claire, had been through the agony of losing her first child shortly after birth. Something that no mother should have to go through. Time had passed and she had been back to the local cemetery to lay flowers at her son's resting place, when she noticed a small plaque bearing the name "Malcolm Watson". You can imagine the delicate nature of a conversation that starts, "I think I spotted your father".

I was confused and equally upset. Why would his wife have interred his ashes without telling me? Why hadn't I known before now? It took a while to sink in, and when it had, I'd chosen to bury my head in the sand and ignore it as much as I could. Today, however, I was going to see if I could find that plaque for myself.

Earlham cemetery in Norwich is a large place with thousands of people buried, or with their ashes scattered there. I'd rung them the day before to try and confirm if my father was really there. At first it seemed like they were unsure and didn't have any records. I'd begun to feel disappointed when a kind lady from their office rang me back "Was he Malcolm James Watson?" she enquired, and with that I knew he was there.

Having only just left my brother's grave I soon found my nerves returning as I headed over to the much larger Earlham cemetery. I've only ever been to the crematorium for the occasional funeral, so I struggled at first to locate the office that might be able to point me to where my father was. The sun was beating down heavily and a muscular chap was busy mowing one of the many lawns. He had a face that fitted in with his location, kindly yet worn in a way of heavy sorrow. He pointed me in the right direction and soon I was being offered a map and a rough direction of where to head.

It seems as though rather than be interred, my father's ashes had been scattered between two large trees and then a plaque put down in his memory somewhere close by. I thank the staff, look at the map and make my way through the first few walkways and memorial gardens.

It looks so tranquil and beautiful in the bright sunshine. Huge rose gardens and fresh flowers line almost every walkway. Considering the amount of tributes that have been left by friends and families, I'm surprisingly alone today. Just the noise of the mower remains, making the perfect summer background track.

At the office I was told that a plaque should be near the two large trees in the corner of the cemetery. As I walk along there are hundreds of small memorial plaques, I start looking and quickly become frustrated as it feels like finding a needle in a haystack. I sit on a bench feeling like I'll never find him and send a message to Claire to try and gauge where she was when she saw him. She confirms that he was on the side of the gravel path I've been walking, so I begin searching again.

I must have looked at every plaque; every one of them in memory of a husband, wife, brother, sister or just a friend. My eyes rest on one or two as I look at the words conveying sense of family. Walking around in a place as big as this you realise you are not alone with feelings of loss. We all feel it, we all go through it.

Frustration appears again. I'm nearly at the end of the pathway and still I have nothing. In anger I shout quietly "come on dad, bloody show yourself!" Call it coincidence, call it fate or simply the fact there were only a few paces of the path left, but soon enough there he is. A simple black plaque with the words "Loving memories Malcolm James Watson 1943-2006"

I was always much closer to my brother, but tears come flooding out. Tears I hadn't expected at all. In part it's the relief of finding him, but mainly it's just the overwhelming sadness of it all. It says "loving memories", but nothing about who those "loving memories" are from. Nothing about a wife, even if she was the second one, nothing about a sister, nothing about children. It's as though he's been dumped here on his own, no flowers, nothing. I cry again. This is my worst fear, I push people away as I'm scared of hurting them by my death, yet I hate the idea of being forgotten, and my father is suffering that fate.

I unwrap my rose plant and place it close to his memorial. I relax back on the grass and oddly feel as close to my Dad as I have for a very long time. It's as though he needs me, and it's not often he would have said that. I searched for 15 months to find my donor, but my donor lead me here. To family, to home.

I find it hard to leave, but eventually I head off, looking back every few minutes to almost check that he is ok. I promise to make sure he won't be left without flowers again. Today completed, I turn my thoughts to the next day ahead. Tomorrow it will be 20 years since my transplant, and 20 years since my donor's death. I may not know him still, but tomorrow I will remember him at a place I love to be. Dovedale.

It's 4:53am and I'm already awake, and I can feel my chest tighten and the nerves in my stomach echoing my fear with the cacophony of sound it's making. I need sleep, but the heat and humidity is only making things worse and I want to feel strong, emotionally, for the day ahead.

After more fitful sleep I get myself up and dressed and down for a cooked breakfast as supplied by the lovely owner of the Station House Bed & Breakfast. Jennifer is here too, always supporting me every step along my journey, and as usual she offers insightful and thought provoking comments. "My teeth are still coming through" she says in a hushed volume that can still be picked up by the other guests. I'm quick to remind her that this isn't the sort of thing a girl in her twenties should be saying to a 43 year old man.

We finish up our breakfast, pay for our accommodation and get in the car for the five minute drive to Dovedale. The weather is expected to be another record breaker, but as we pull up in the car park, there is a smattering of rain. After much debate we both pack some waterproofs along with a supply of sun tan lotion. Good old Britain, you need everything on days like this.

Dovedale is a small valley that the river Dove winds through. Owned by the National Trust, there is a walkway running for 3 miles between Thorpe Cloud and Milldale. I've come here many times just to enjoy the beautiful scenery, and it's something I always enjoy, so when I decided I needed a place to remember my donor, it seemed the obvious choice. In my head I hope my heart has been here before many years ago as well. I want it to mean something.

We put all our things into one small backpack and Jennifer takes the bunch of white roses mixed with carnations that I've brought along to place in memory of my unknown donor, and whose family I know will be grieving today. As we start the wind picks up and rain begins to fall. This isn't how it was meant to be, I was hoping for glorious sunshine.

Soon we are upon Dovedale's famous stepping stones that cross the river, and normally people stop here to take a photo, leaving other crossers patiently waiting the other side. Today, however, Jennifer and I are alone yet we don't stop. We quickly carry on in search of a break from the wind.

I already have in my mind where I want to leave my flowers, and it's something I hope could become an annual event with other transplantees or donor families joining me. The site is a place called "Lovers Leap". Whilst it sounds slightly morbid, the girl who supposedly threw herself from the limestone rock, 120 foot above the river, survived her fall by landing in some thick bushes. Her reason for jumping was being jilted by her lover, yet on survival she remained happy and single for the rest of her life.

As we climb the path to approach "Lovers Leap" we are bathed in glorious and warm sunshine. So much so I already begin to struggle as I make the last few steps. We both stop at a bench viewing the rocks, and agree this is the right place to leave the flowers, but before I do I just really want a moment's reflection on what's brought me here.

These past 15 months have been some of the most difficult of my life. That might seem overly dramatic for someone that has been through the grief of losing a brother, and also the stresses of transplantation, but I was always fighting back then. The fight feels knocked out of me now.

People always see me as a survivor, someone who just laughs and enjoys life, and gets on with things as best he can, but the truth is I've always had to cope. Cope with thoughts about death. Thoughts about my donor and brother. Thoughts about surviving when others lose that battle. I'm tired though, tired of coping and in need of a long rest.

Through my writing I've learned that most of the transplant patients I speak to have to cope too. So do the donor families who mean so much to us. We are all dealing with our own history, our own battles, but it seems we really are in this together.

A transplant is far from a cure, but it extends life, and for that we are lucky to have so many health care professionals with our interests at heart. Life can only be extended by the loss of another, and that's the biggest miracle that donation brings. One family, in their weakest and darkest moment, reaches out and offers light to another. Light to someone they don't even know.

As I've struggled through the emotional wreckage of my writing, I've sometimes felt it was time to let the journey end. To switch off life and put an end to an energy that feels drained and unable to go again. Life has been given to me though, not just once but twice and whilst I might not know my donor, I feel closer to him today than I ever have done before. I know him.

I can't tell you if cellular memory exists, but I haven't met anyone, transplantee or donor family that hasn't wanted that connection. The love and compassion between recipients and families runs deeper than any relationship I know, and helps promote organ donation to those who hopefully will never be in our position. What Claire Sylvia did, was simply bring that relationship out into the open, and voice what nearly all patients think. We love our donors.

Sylvia's daughter Amara said "If you can, try and find out about your donor, if nothing else it will bring closure to you."

I may not know him as much as I'd like, but I've spent the last 15 months thinking about nothing else, and I've felt his presence grow and take form in both my mind and my heart. I don't have that name or a photo, but what I have is beautiful and unique.

I make my way up the small outcrop of rock that's in front of me, and lay my flowers at its crest. The sunshine lighting up the white petals of the six roses. An amazing gift was given, life extended and it's a life I know I can continue to love.

For my donor.

12251570R00182

Printed in Great Britain
by Amazon.co.uk, Ltd.,
Marston Gate.